1

OCCULT PRINCIPLES OF HEALTH AND HEALING

By MAX HEINDEL

FOREWORD

This compilation of material concerning the health and healing of the human organism as considered from the occult viewpoint affords those interested in attaining and maintaining health a treasure chest of valuable information. Max Heindel, a trained clairvoyant and investigator of the super-physical worlds, devoted much time and effort to ascertaining the real causes of physical and mental disorders as revealed in the realm of cause, the higher or superphysical planes, and this volume contains the fruits of his labor. It embodies some of the most priceless truths in regard to the origin, functions, and proper care of the vehicles of man to be found on the printed page, and those concerned with the true art of healing will find it an indispensable addition to their libraries.

Christ admonished His disciples: "Preach the Gospel, and heal the sick." Maintaining health, when once gained or regained, requires a knowledge of "the Gospel," or laws of God, and it is therefore in the light of both parts of the command of the Great Teacher that this book is dedicated to the afflicted of humanity. May the contents of its pages, permeated as they are with the love and compassionate understanding of the mystic heart of the author, be the means of bringing new solace and relief to countless aching hearts and suffering bodies, as well as speed the day for the generation of more perfect human vehicles.

CONTENTS

PLATES

PART I

MAN AND HIS VEHICLES

CHAPTER I

THE DENSE BODY

INTRODUCTION:

Occult science teaches that man is a complex being who possesses:

(1) A DENSE BODY, which is the visible instrument he uses here in this world to fetch and carry; the body we ordinarily think of as the whole man.

(2) A VITAL BODY, which is made of ether and pervades the visible body as ether permeates all other forms, except that human beings specialize a greater amount of the universal ether than other forms. That ethereal body is our instrument for specializing the vital energy of the Sun.

(3) A DESIRE BODY, which is our emotional nature. This finer vehicle pervades both the vital and dense bodies. It is seen by clairvoyant vision to extend about sixteen inches outside our visible body, which is located in the center of this ovoid cloud as the yolk is in the center of the egg.

(4) THE MIND, which is a mirror, reflecting the outer world and enabling the Ego to transmit its commands as thought and word, also to compel action.

The Ego is the threefold Spirit which uses these vehicles to gather experience in the school of life.

EVOLUTION:

The dense body was the first vehicle built and has therefore an enormous period of evolution back of it. It is in its fourth stage of development and has now reached a great and marvelous degree of efficiency. It will, in time, reach perfection, but even at present it is the best organized of man's vehicles. It is a wonderfully constructed instrument and should be recognized as such by everyone pretending to have any knowledge of the constitution of man.

The germ of the dense body was given by the Lords of Flame during the first Revolution of the Saturn Period, the first of the Seven Great Days of Manifestation according to the Rosicrucian Teachings. This germ was somewhat developed during the remainder of the first six Revolutions, being given the capacity for developing the sense organs, particularly the ear. Therefore, the ear is the most highly developed organ we possess.

In the first half of the Saturn Revolution of the Sun Period, the second of the Seven Great Days of Manifestation, the Lords of Flame were concerned with certain improvements to be made upon the germ of the dense body. It became necessary to change the germ in such a way as to allow of interpenetration by a vital body, also capability of evolving glands and an alimentary canal. This was done by the joint action of the Lords of Flame and the Lords of Wisdom.

In the first or Saturn Revolution of the Moon Period, the third of the Seven Great Days of Manifestation, the Lords of Wisdom cooperated with the Lords of Individuality to reconstruct the germ of the dense body. This germ had unfolded embryonic sense organs, digestive organs, glands, etc. and was interpenetrated by a budding vital body. Of course, it was not solid and visible as it is now, yet in a crude sort of way it was somewhat organized. In the Moon Period it was necessary to reconstruct it and make it capable of being interpenetrated by a desire body, and also capable of evolving a nervous system, muscle, cartilage, and a rudimentary skeleton. This reconstruction was the work of the Saturn Revolution of the Moon Period. These Moon beings were not so purely germinal as in the previous periods. To the trained clairvoyant they appear suspended by strings in the atmosphere of the fire-fog, as the embryo hangs from the placenta by the umbilical cord. Currents, which provided some sort of nourishment, flowed in and out from the atmosphere through those cords.

When the Earth came out of chaos, at the beginning of the Earth period, it was at first in the dark red stage known as the Polarian Epoch. There humanity first evolved a DENSE BODY, the germ of which was given by the lords of Flame during the First Revolution of the Saturn Period. It was not then at all like our present vehicle, of course. When the condition of the Earth became fiery, as in the Hyperborean Epoch, the VITAL BODY was added and man became plant-like, that is to say, he had the same vehicles as our plants have today, and also a similar consciousness, or rather, unconsciousness, to that which we have in dreamless sleep when the DENSE and VITAL bodies are left upon the bed.

At that time, in the Hyperborean Epoch, the body of man was like an enormous gas bag, floating outside the fiery Earth, and it threw off plant-like spores, which then grew and were used by other incoming entities. At that time man was double sexed, a hermaphrodite.

In the Lemurian Epoch, when the Earth had somewhat cooled and islands of crust had begun to form amid boiling seas, then also man's body had somewhat solidified and had become more like the body we see today. It was apelike, a short trunk with enormous arms and limbs, the heels projecting backward, and almost no head--at least the upper part of the head was nearly entirely wanting. Man lived in the atmosphere of steam which occultists called fire-fog, and had no lungs, but breathed by means of tubes. He had the gill-like apparatus still present in the human embryo while passing through the stage of antenatal life corresponding to that epoch. He had no warm, red blood, for at that stage there was no individual Spirit. He had a bladder-like organ inside, which he inflated with heated air to help him leap enormous chasms when volcanic eruptions destroyed the land upon which he was living. From the back of his head there projected an organ which has now drawn into the head and is called by anatomists the PINEAL GLAND, or the third eye, although it was never an eye, but a localized organ of feeling. The body was then devoid of feeling, but when man came too close to a volcanic crater, the heat was registered by this organ to warn him away before his body was destroyed.

At that time the body had already so far solidified that it was impossible for man to continue to propagate by spores, and it was necessary that he should evolve an organ of thought, a brain. The creative force which we now use to build railways, steamships, etc., in the outer world, was then used inwardly for the building of organs. Like all forces it was positive and negative. One pole was turned upward to build the brain, leaving the other pole available for the creation of another body. Thus man was no longer a complete creative unit. Each possessed only half the creative force, and it was therefore necessary for him to seek his complement outside himself.

In the latter part of the Lemurian Epoch the form of man was yet quite plastic. The skeleton had formed, but man himself had great power in molding the flesh of his own body, and that of the animals about him.

At this time, when he was born, man could hear and feel, but his perception of light came later. The Lemurian had no eyes. He had two sensitive spots which were affected by the light of the sun as it shone dimly through the fiery atmosphere of ancient Lemuria, but it was not until nearly the close of the Atlantean Epoch that he had sight as we have it today.

His language consisted of sounds like those of Nature. The sighing of the wind in the immense forests which grew in great luxuriance in that super-tropical climate, the rippling of the brook, the howling of the tempest, the thunder of the waterfall, the roar of the volcano--all these were to him voices of the Gods from whom he knew himself to have descended.

Of the birth of his body he knew nothing. He could not SEE either it or anything else, but he did PERCEIVE his fellow beings. It was, however, an inner perception, like our perception of persons and things in dreams, but with this very important difference, that his dream-perception was clear and rational.

But when "their eyes were opened" (as told in the story of the "Fall") and their consciousness was directed outward towards the facts of the physical World, conditions were altered. Propagation was directed, not by Angels, but by man, who was ignorant of the operation of the Sun- and Moon-forces. His consciousness became focused in the Physical World, although things did not appear to his vision with clearly defined outlines until the latter part of the Atlantean Epoch. Still he came by degrees to know death because of the break made in his consciousness when it was shifted to the higher worlds at death and back to the Physical World at rebirth.

However, what has been said about the enlightenment of the Lemurians applies to only a minor portion of those who lived in the latter part of that epoch, and who became the seed for the seven Atlantean Races. The greater part of the Lemurians were animal-like and the FORMS inhabited by them have degenerated into the savages and anthropoids of the present day.

In the Atlantean Epoch, which followed the Lemurian, man was very different from anything existent on Earth at the present time. He had a head, but scarcely any forehead, his brain had no frontal development; the head sloped almost abruptly back from a point just above the eyes. As compared with our present humanity, he was a giant; his arms and legs were much longer in proportion to his body than ours. Instead of walking, he progressed by a series of flying leaps, not unlike those of the kangaroo. He had small blinking eyes and his hair was round in section. The latter peculiarity, if no other, distinguishes the descendants of the Atlantean Races who remain with us at the present time. Their hair was straight, glossy, black and round in section. That of the Aryan, though it may differ in color, is always OVAL in section. The ears of the Atlantean sat much farther back upon the head than do those of the Aryan.

The higher vehicles of the early Atlanteans were not drawn into a concentric position in relation to the dense body, as are ours. The Spirit was not quite an indwelling Spirit; it was partially outside, therefore could not control its vehicles with as great facility as though it dwelt entirely inside. The head of the vital body was outside of and held a position far above the physical head. There is a point between the eyebrows and about half an inch below the surface of the skin, which has a corresponding point in the vital body. When these two points come into correspondence, as they do in man today, they form the seat of the indwelling Spirit in the man.

On account of the distance between these two points, the Atlantean's powers of perception or vision was much keener in the inner worlds than in the dense Physical World, obscured by its atmosphere of thick, heavy fog. In the fullness of time, however, the atmosphere slowly became clearer; at the same time, the point spoken of in the vital body came closer and closer to the corresponding point in the dense body, being united to it in the last third of the Atlantean Epoch.

The Rmoahals were the first of the Atlantean Races. They had but little memory and that little was connected with sensations. They remembered colors and tones, and thus to some extent they evolved Feeling. With memory came to the Atlanteans the rudiments of a language. They evolved words and no longer made use of mere sounds, as did the Lemurians, giving names to things.

The Tlavatlis were the second Atlantean Race. Already they began to feel their worth as separate human beings. They became ambitious; the demanded that their works be remembered. Memory became a factor in the life of the community. Thus began ancestor worship.

The Toltecs were the third Atlantean Race. They inaugurated Monarchy and Hereditary Succession, originating the custom of honoring men for the deeds done by their ancestors. Experience came to be highly valued, and memory was developed to a very great degree.

In the middle third of Atlantis we find the beginning of separate nations. In the time the Kings became intoxicated with power, and began to use their power corruptly, for selfish ends and personal aggrandizement instead of for the common good.

The Original Turanians were the fourth Atlantean Race. They were especially vile in their abominable selfishness, erecting temples where the Kings were worshiped as Gods.

The Original Semites were the fifth and most important of the seven Atlantean Races, because in them we find the first germ of the corrective quality of thought. Therefore the Original Semitic Race became the "seed-race" for the seven races of the Aryan Epoch. They were the first to discover that "brain" is superior to "brawn." During the existence of this race, the atmosphere of Atlantic commenced to clear definitely, and the previously mentioned point in the vital body came into correspondence with its companion point in the dense body. The combination of events gave man the ability to see objects clearly with sharp, well-defined contours; but it also resulted in loss of the sight pertaining to the inner worlds.

The Akkadians were the sixth and the Mongolians were the seventh of the Atlantean Races. They evolved the faculty of thought still farther, but followed lines of reasoning which deviated more and more from the main trend of the developing life. As the heavy fogs of Atlantis condensed more and more, the increasing quantity of water gradually inundated that continent, destroying the greater part of the population and the evidences of their civilization.

Central Asia was the cradle of the Aryan Races, who descended from the original Semites. Thence have the different races gone out. It is unnecessary to describe them here, as historical researches have sufficiently revealed their main features.

THE BRAIN AND NERVOUS SYSTEMS:

In the Saturn Revolution of the Earth period the dense body was given the ability to form a brain and become a vehicle for the germ of mind which was to be added later. The impulse was given to building the frontal part of the brain. The brain and the nervous systems are the highest expression of the desire body. They call up pictures of the outside world, but in mental image-making, the blood brings the material for the pictures; therefore, when thought is active the blood flows to the head.

In man the brain is the link between the Spirit and the outside world. He can know nothing of the outside world except through the medium of the brain. The sense organs are merely carriers to the brain of impacts from without and the brain is the instrument which interprets and coordinates those impacts. The Spirit, aided by the Angels, built the brain to gather knowledge of the Physical World. When the Ego entered into possession of its vehicles it became necessary to use part of the creative force for the building of a brain and larynx. The Lucifers are the instigators of all mental activity, by means of the part of the sex force that is carried upward for work in the brain. Thus did the evolving entity obtain brain consciousness of the outside world at the cost of half its creative power.

Physiologists note that certain areas of the brain are devoted to particular thought activities, and phrenologists have carried this branch of science still farther. Now, it is known that thought breaks down and destroys nerve tissues. This and all other waste of the body, is replaced by the blood. When, through the development of the heart into a voluntary muscle, the circulation of the blood finally passes under the absolute control of the unifying Life Spirit it will then be within the power of that Spirit to withhold the blood from those areas of the mind devoted to selfish purposes. As a result, those particular thought centers will gradually atrophy.

Brain-knowledge, with its concomitant selfishness, was bought by man at the cost of the power to create from himself alone. He bought his free will at the cost of pain and death; but when man learns to use his intellect for the good of humanity, he will gain spiritual power over life, and in addition, will be guided by an innate knowledge as much higher than the present brain-consciousness as that is higher than the lowest animal consciousness. The brain is, at best, only an indirect way of gaining knowledge and will be superseded by direct touch with the Wisdom of Nature, which man, without any cooperation, will then be able to use for the creation of new bodies.

In the Moon Period it was necessary to reconstruct the dense body to make it capable of being interpenetrated by a desire body, and also capable of evolving a nervous system, muscle, cartilage, and a rudimentary skeleton. This reconstruction was the work of the Saturn Revolution of the Moon Period.

The reconstruction of the dense body in the Saturn Revolution of the Earth Period gave the first impulse to the incipient division in the nervous system which has since become apparent in its subdivisions: the voluntary and the sympathetic. The latter was the only one provided for in the Moon Period. The voluntary nervous system (which has transformed the dense body from a mere automaton acting under stimuli from without, to an extraordinary adaptable instrument capable of being guided and controlled by an Ego from within) was not added until the present Earth Period.

When the division of the Sun, Moon, and Earth took place, in the early part of the Lemurian Epoch, the more advanced portion of humanity-in-the-making experienced a division of the desire body into a higher and a lower part. The reset of humanity did likewise in the early part of the Atlantean Epoch. This higher part of the desire body became a sort of animal soul. It built the cerebrospinal nervous system and the voluntary muscles, by that means controlling the lower part of the threefold body until the link of mind was given.

Part of the involuntary muscular system is controlled by the sympathetic nervous system.

The seat of the Human Spirit is primarily in the pineal gland and secondarily in the brain and the cerebrospinal nervous system, which controls the voluntary muscles.

THE BLOOD:

The study of the blood is very deep, far-reaching, and of supreme importance from whatever viewpoint we analyze it. Lucifer was decidedly right when he said that "blood is a most peculiar essence." It builds the physical body from the time the seed atom is deposited in the ovum till he rupture of the silver cord ends material existence, being one of the highest products of the vital body and the carrier of nourishment to every part of the body. It is the direct vehicle of the Ego, having injected into it every thought, feeling or emotion transmitted to the lungs.

In infancy, and up to the fourteenth year, the red marrow-bones do not make all the blood corpuscles. Most of them are supplied by the thymus gland, which is largest in the fetus and gradually diminishes as the individual blood-making faculty develops in the growing child. The thymus gland contains, as it were, a supply of blood corpuscles given by the parents, and consequently the child, which draws its blood from that source, does not realize its individuality. Not until the blood is made by the child does it think of itself as "I," and when the thymus gland disappears, at the age of fourteen, the "I" feeling reaches its full expression, for then the blood is made and dominated entirely by the Ego. The following will make clear the idea and its logic:

It will be remembered that assimilation and growth depend upon the forces working along the positive pole of the vital body's chemical ether. That is set free at the seventh year, together with the balance of the vital body. Only the chemical ether is fully ripe at that time; the other parts need more ripening. At the fourteenth year the life ether of the vital body, which has to do with propagation, is fully ripe. In the period from seven to fourteen years of age the excessive assimilation has stored an amount of fore which goes to the sex organs and is ready at the time the desire body is set free.

This force of sex is stored in the blood during the third of the seven year periods and in that time the light ether, which is the avenue for the blood heat, is developed and controls the heart, so that the body is neither too hot nor too cold. In early childhood the blood very often rises to an abnormal temperature. During the period of excessive growth, it is frequently the reverse, but in the hot-headed, unrestrained youth, passion and temper very often drive the Ego out by overheating the blood. We very appropriately call this an ebullition or boiling over of temper and describe the effect as causing the person to "lose his head," or become incapable of thought. That is exactly what happens when passion, rage, or temper overheats the blood, thus drawing the Ego outside the bodies. The Ego is outside of its vehicles and they are running as much, bereft of the guiding influence of thought, part of the work of which is to act as a brake on impulse. Only the man who keeps cool and does not allow excess of heat to drive him out can think properly.

As proof of the assertion that the Ego cannot work in the body when the blood is either too hot or too cold we will call attention to the well-known fact that excessive heat makes one sleepy, and, if carried beyond a certain point, it drives the Ego out, leaving the body unconscious. It is only when the blood is at or near the normal temperature that the Ego can use it as a vehicle of consciousness.

The burnish blush of shame is an evidence of the manner in which the blood is driven to the head, thus overheating the brain and paralyzing thought. Fear is a state when the Ego wants to barricade himself against some outside danger. He then drives the blood to the center and grows pale, because the blood has left the periphery of the body, and has lost heat, thus paralyzing thought. In fever the excess of heat causes delirium.

The full-blooded person, though the blood is not too hot, is active in body and mind, while the anemic person is sleepy. In one the Ego has better control; in the other, less. When the Ego wants to think it drives blood, at the proper heat, to the brain. When a heavy meal centers the activity of the Ego upon the digestive tract, the man cannot think; he is sleepy.

The old Norsemen and the Scots recognized that the Ego is in the blood. No stranger could become associated with them as a relative until he had "mixed blood" with them and thus become one of them.

In the descendants of the patriarchal families--Adam, Methuselah, etc., the blood which coursed through their veins contained the pictures of all that had happened to their different ancestors, and these pictures were constantly before the inner vision of each one as they had no outer vision at that time. At the present time the blood of each individual contains only the pictures of his own individual experiences and the subconscious mind has access to them. Up to the time that marriage outside of the family was commenced individuals were ruled by a Family Spirit (Angel) which entered the blood by means of the air inspired, and helped each Ego to control its vehicles. When marriage outside the family began, Egos had arrived at a point in the evolution of self-consciousness where they could depend on self, and where they were to ease being God-guided automatons and become self-governing individuals. The greater the mixture of blood the less the indwelling Ego can be influenced by the Race or Family Spirits. Unmixed blood gave us ancestral assistance when we needed it. Mixed blood makes for independence of outside help. A God (creator) must be independent.

The heat of the blood is the vantage ground of the Ego, and the Lucifer Spirits from Mars aid in maintaining this heat by dissolving iron, a Mars metal, in our blood to attract oxygen, a solar element.

The proper heat for the real expression of the Ego is not present until the mind is born from the macrocosmic Concrete Mind, when the individual is about twenty-one years old. Statutory law also recognizes this as the earliest age when the man is deemed fit to exercise a franchise.

In the lower order of animals blood is fluid and nucleated. The nuclei, enters of life, are the vantage ground of a Group Spirit. It regulates their vital processes and guides them through the nuclei. During the early part of the gestatory period the blood of the fetus is also nucleated by the life of the mother, and she regulates the process of body building, but as soon as the incoming Ego enters the mothers body, it commences to assert its individuality and resists formation of nucleated blood cells. The old cells gradually disappear, so that when the silver cord is tied at the time of quickening and the Ego is drawn into its body, all nuclei have disappeared, and it is absolute autocrat of its new vehicle, a heritage more precious than any other earthly possession; and when properly used it is our means of generating soul power and laying up treasure in heaven. When we abandon this vehicle to Spirit controls, we seriously hinder our higher evolution and commit a great sin.

Thus the blood is the particular vehicle of the Ego, and as in the past eons of development we have crystallized matter in order to form our dense body, so also it is destined that now we must etherealize our vehicles in order that we may lift ourselves and the world out of the realms of materiality and into the spiritual. Naturally, therefore, the Ego aims first to make the blood gaseous, and to the spiritual sight, this red unnucleated blood is not a fluid, but a gas. It is no argument against this assertion that the moment we prick our skin the blood comes out as a liquid. The moment we open up the try-cock of a steam boiler the gas also condenses into a liquid, but if we make a model steam engine of glass and look at the way steam works there we shall see only the piston move backward and forward, driven by an invisible agent, LIVE STEAM, and similarly, as the live steam direct from the boiler is invisible, and gaseous, so also the LIVE BLOOD in the human body is a gas, and the higher the state of development of any given Ego, the more ethereal is it able to make the blood.

When, by the vital processes, food has reached the highest alchemical state, the process of condensation begins and the blood-gas is formed into tissue in the various organs to replace what has been wasted or destroyed by the activities of the body. The spleen is the gateway of the vital body; there the solar force which abounds in the surrounding atmosphere enters in a constraint stream, to aid us in the vital processes, and there also the war between the desire body and the vital body is waged most fiercely. Thoughts of worry, fear, and anger interfere with the process of evaporation in the spleen, a speck of plasm is the result, and this is at once seized upon by a thought elemental which forms a nucleus and embodies itself therein. Then it commences to live a life of destruction, coalescing with other waste products and decaying elements wherever formed, making the body a charnel house instead of the temple of in indwelling living Spirit. We may therefore say EVERY WHITE CORPUSCLE WHICH HAS BEEN TAKEN BY AN OUTSIDE ENTITY IS TO THE EGO A LOST OPPORTUNITY. The more of these lost opportunities there are in the body, the less is the body under control of the Ego, therefore we find them present in larger numbers in all diseases than when the person is in health. It may also be said that the person of jovial good nature or one who is devoutly religious and has an absolute faith and trust in divine providence and love, will register many less lost opportunities or white corpuscles than those who are always worrying and fretting.

So it is that the blood is the only part of the body really course. The measure in which we control all blood depends upon the Ego's ability to express itself through the body. It is only through the red corpuscles that the Ego is able to work. Whenever we allow ourselves to be negative we manufacture white corpuscles, which are not, as we have seen, "the policemen of the system," as science now thinks, but destroyers.

When the blood courses through the arteries which are deep in the body, it is a gas, as has been shown; but loss of heat near the surface of the body causes it to partially condense, and in that substance the Ego is learning to form mineral crystals. Science has lately found that the blood of different people has different crystals, so that it is possible now to the tell the blood of a Negro from the blood of a white man; but there will come a day when they will know a still greater difference; for just as there is a difference in the crystals formed by the different races, so there is also a difference in the crystals formed by each individual man.

Looking at the matter from another angle, we may note that when blood is beaten with a stick it separates into three distinct substances: the serum or water-like substance which comes under Cancer ruled by the Moon (Lunar Hierarchy); the red coloring matter which is the Martian substance generated under Scorpio; and most important of all, the fibrin, or stringy matter which is under the third of the watery signs, Pisces. When the skeleton was outside our flesh, consciousness was dull as in the crustacea. By getting outside the bony structure we have gained a much higher grade of consciousness, and by spiritualizing this inner skeleton through the medium of the blood, we extract the essence of all we have learned in the past epochs and transform it to usable soul power in the Jupiter Period. To interfere in this work is a crime against the soul.

Since woman has the positive vital body, she matures earlier than the male, and the parts which remain plant-like, such as the hair, grow longer and more luxuriant. Naturally positive vital body will generate more blood than the negative vital body possessed by the male, hence we have in woman a greater blood pressure, which it is necessary to relieve by the periodical flow, and when that eases at the climacteric period there is a second growth in woman, particularly well expressed in the saying, "fat and forty."

The impulses of the desire body drive the blood through the system at varying rates of speed, according to the strength of the emotions. Woman, having an excess of blood, works under much higher pressure than man, and while this pressure is relieved by the periodical flow, there are times when it is necessary to have an extra outlet; then the tears of woman, which are WHITE BLEEDING, act as a safety valve to remove the excessive fluid. Men, although they may have as strong emotions as women, are not given to tears because they have no more blood than they can comfortably use.

The blood is now differently constituted from what it was in the earlier ages of human evolution. The Christ Spirit was seen at the Baptism to descent upon Jesus' body. Jesus himself, the Spirit, left that body and was given a mission to serve the churches while his body was being used for direct teaching by the Christ, and his blood was being prepared as an OPEN SESAME to the Kingdom of God.

When anyone is killed, the Venus blood with its impurities clings closely to the flesh, and therefore the arterial blood which flows is distinctly leaner than it would otherwise be. Being etherealized by the great Christ Spirit, the cleansed blood of Jesus overflowed the world, purified the Etheric Region of selfishness to a great extent, and gave man a better chance to draw to himself materials which will allow him to form altruistic purposes and desires.

THE DUCTLESS GLANDS:

It is well known to the esoteric astrologer that the human body has an immense period of evolution behind it and that this splendid organism is the result of a slow process of gradual upbuilding which is still continuing and will make each generation better than the previous until in some far distant future it shall have reached a stage of completion of which we cannot even dream. It is also understood by the deeper students that in addition to the physical body man has finer vehicles which are not yet seen by the great majority of human beings, though all have within them latent a sixth sense whereby they will in time cognize these finer sheaths of the soul.

The occultist speaks of these finer vehicles as the vital body, made of ether, and the desire body, made of desire stuff, the material whence we draw our feelings and emotions, and with the addition of the SHEATH OF MIND and the physical body these complete what may be termed the personality which is the evanescent part distinct from the immortal Spirit that uses these vehicles for its expression. These finer vehicles interpenetrate the dense physical body as air permeates water and have particular dominion over certain parts thereof, because the physical body itself is a crystallization of these finer vehicles in the same manner and upon the same principle that the soft fluids of a snail's body gradually crystallize into the hard and flinty shell which it carries upon its back. For the purpose of this dissertation we may say broadly that the softer parts of our bodies which we commonly call flesh may be divided into two kinds, glands and muscles.

The vital body was started in the Sun Period. Crystallization from that time on it that vehicle has developed what we now call glands and to this day they and the blood are the special manifestations of the vital body within the physical vehicle. Therefore, the glands as a whole may be said to be under the rule of the life-giving Sun and the great benefic, Jupiter. It is the function of the vital body to build and restore the tone of the muscles when tense and tired by the work imposed upon them by the restless desire body, which was started in the Moon Period. The muscles are therefore ruled by the wandering Moon, which is the present vantage point of the Angels, the humanity of the Moon period, and by the impulsive and turbulent Mars, where the so-called "Fallen Angels," the Lucifer Spirits, dwell. That is to say, as a whole, for the student must carefully note that individual glands and particular groups of muscles are under the rulership of other planets as well. It is as when we say that all who live in the United States of America are citizens of that country, but some are subject to the laws of California, others to those of Maine, etc.

We know the Hermetic Axiom, "As above, so below," which is the master key to all mysteries, and as there are upon the Earth, the macrocosm, a great many undiscovered places, so also in the microcosm of the body do we find unknown countries that are a closed book to the scientific explorers. Chief among them has been a small group of the so-called "ductless glands," seven in number, namely:

The Pituitary Body, ruled by Uranus.

The Pineal Gland, ruled by Neptune.

The Thyroid Gland, ruled by Mercury.

The Thymus Gland, ruled by Venus.

The Spleen, ruled by the Sun.

The two Adrenals, ruled by Jupiter.

They have a great and particular interest for occultists, and they may be termed in a certain sense "the seven roses" upon the Cross of the body, for they are intimately connected with the occult development of humanity. Four of them, the thymus gland, the spleen, and the two adrenals are connected with the personality. The pituitary body and the pineal gland are particularly correlated with the spiritual side of our nature and the thyroid gland forms the link between. The astrological rulership is as follows:

The spleen is the entrance gate of the solar forces specialized by each human being and circulated through the body as the vital fluid, without which no being can live. This organ is therefore governed by the Sun. The two adrenals are under the rulership of Jupiter, the great benefic, and exert a calming, quieting and soothing effect when the emotional activities of the

Moon and Mars or Saturn have destroyed the poise. When the obstructive hand of Saturn has awakened the melancholy emotions and laid its restraint upon the heart, the adrenals' secretions are carried by the blood to the heart and act as a powerful stimulant in its effort to keep up the circulation, while the jovial optimism struggles against the saturnine worries or against the impulse of Mars, which stirs the desire body into turbulent emotions of anger, rendering the muscles tense and trembling, dissipating the energy of the system. Then the secretion of the adrenals comes to the rescue, releasing the glycogen of the liver in a more abundant measure than usual to cope with the emergency until the equipoise has been again attained, and similarly during whatever other stress or strain. It was the knowledge of this occult fact that prompted the ancient astrologers to place the kidneys under the rulership of Libra, the Balance, and in order to avoid confusion of ideas we may say that the kidneys themselves play an important part in the nutrition of the body, being under the rulership of Venus, the Lady of Libra. However, Jupiter governs the adrenals, with which we are now particularly engaged.

Both Venus and her higher octave, Uranus, govern the functions of nutrition and growth, but in different ways and for different purposes. Therefore Venus rules the thymus gland, which is the link between the parents and the child until the latter has reached puberty. This gland is located immediately behind the sternum or breast bone. It is largest in antenatal life and through childhood while growth is excessive and rapid. During that time the vital body of the child does its most effective work, for the child is not then subject to the passions and emotions generated by the desire body after that comes to birth at or about the fourteenth year. But during the years of growth the child cannot manufacture the red blood corpuscles as does the adult, for the unborn, unorganized desire body does not then act as an avenue for the martian forces which assimilate the iron from the food and transmute it into hemoglobin. To compensate for this lack there is stored in the thymus gland a spiritual essence drawn from the parents, and with this essence provided by their love the child is able to accomplish the alchemistry of blood temporarily until its desire body becomes dynamically active. Then the thymus gland atrophies and the child draws from its own desire body the necessary martian force. From that time, under normal conditions, Uranus, the octave of Venus, and ruler of the pituitary body, takes charge of the function of growth and assimilation in the following manner.

It is well known that all things, our food included, radiate from themselves continuously small particles which given an index of the thing whence they emanate, its quality included. Thus when we lift the food to our mouth a number of these invisible particles enter the nose and by excitation of the olfactory tract convey to us a knowledge whether the food we are about to take is suitable for this purpose or not, the sense of smell warning us to discard such foods as have a noxious odor, etc. But besides those particles which attract or repel us from food by their action on the olfactory tract through the sense of smell, there are others which penetrate the sphenoid bone, impinge upon the pituitary body and start the Uranian alchemistry by which a secretion is formed and injected into the blood. This furthers assimilation through the chemical ether, thus affecting the normal growth and well-being of the human body through life. Sometimes this Uranian influence of the pituitary body is eccentric and therefore responsible for strange and abnormal growths which produce the unfortunate freaks of Nature we occasionally meet.

But besides being responsible for the spiritual impulses which generate the before-mentioned physical manifestations of growth, Uranus, working through the pituitary body, is also responsible for the spiritual phases of growth which aid awakened man in his efforts to penetrate the veil into the invisible worlds. In this work it is, however, associated with Neptune, the ruler of the pineal gland, and it will therefore be necessary, in order to properly elucidate, that we study the functions of the thyroid gland, ruled by Mercury, and of the pineal gland which is under the domination of his higher octave, Neptune, simultaneously.

That the thyroid gland is under the rule of Mercury, the planet of reason, is readily realized when we understand the effect which the degeneration of this gland has upon the mind, as shown in the diseases of Cretinism and Myxedema. The secretions of this gland are as necessary to the proper functioning of the mind as ether is to the transmission of electricity, that is to say, upon the physical plane of existence where the brain transmutes thought into action. Contact with and expression in the invisible worlds depends upon the functional ability of the pineal gland, which is altogether spiritual and is therefore ruled by the octave of Mercury, Neptune, the planet of spirituality, which operates in conjunction with the pituitary body ruled by Uranus.

Scientists have wasted much time in speculation upon the nature and function of these two little bodies, the pituitary body and the pineal gland, but without avail, and principally because, as Mephistopheles says so sarcastically to the young man who wants to study science under Faust:

"WHO E'ER WOULD KNOW AND TREAT OF AUGHT ALIVE

SEEKS FIRST THE LIVING SPIRIT THENCE TO DRIVE;

THEN ARE THE LIFELESS FRAGMENTS IN HIS HAND;

HE LACKS, ALAS! THE VITAL SPIRIT BAND."

No one can really and truly observe the physiological functions of any organ under such conditions as exist in the laboratory, on the operating table, or in the dissection or vivisection chamber. To arrive at an adequate understanding one must necessarily see these organs exercising their physiological functions IN THE LIVING BODY, and that can only be done by means of spiritual sight. There are a number of organs which are either atrophying or developing; the former show the path we have already traveled during our past evolution, the latter are finger posts, indicating our future development. But there is still another class of organs which are neither degenerating nor evolving; they are simply dormant (spiritually) at the present time. Physiologists believe that the pituitary body and the pineal gland are atrophying because they find these organs more developed in some of the lower classes of life, such as worms, but as a matter of fact they are wrong in their ideas. Some have also suspected that the pineal gland is in some way connected with the mind, because it contains certain crystals after death, and the quantity was much less in those who were mentally defective than in people of normal mentality. This conclusion is right, but the Seer knows that the spinal canal of the living is not filled with

FLUID; that the blood is not LIQUID, and that these organs have no crystals in them when the body is alive.

These assertions are made with full knowledge of the fact that the blood and the spinal essence are liquid when drawn out of the body, living or dead, and the contents of the pituitary body and the pineal gland APPEAR crystalline when the brain is dissected. However, the reason is similar to that which causes steam drawn from a steam boiler to condense immediately upon contact with the atmosphere, and molten metal drawn from a smelter's furnace to crystallize immediately upon withdrawal therefrom.

All these substances are purely spiritual essences when inside the body; they are then ethereal and the substance in the pineal gland, when seen by the spiritual sight, appears as LIGHT. Furthermore, when one Seer looks upon the pineal gland of another who is then also exercising his spiritual faculties, this light is of a most intense brilliancy and of an iridescence similar to but transcending in beauty the most wonderful play of the Northern Lights, the AURORA BOREALIS. It may also be said that the function of this organ seems to have changed in the course of human evolution. During the earlier epochs of our present stay upon the Earth, when man's body was a large, baggy thing into which the Spirit had not yet entered, but was there only as an overshadowing presence, there was an opening in the top and the pineal gland was within it. It was then an organ of orientation, giving a sense of direction. As the human body condensed, it became less and less able to endure the intense heat which prevailed during that time and the pineal gland gave warning when the body was brought too near one of the many raters and active volcanoes which were then erupting the thin Earth crust, thus enabling the Spirit to guide it away from these dangerous places. It was an organ of direction which operated by feeling, but feeling has since been distributed over the skin of the whole body. This is an indication to the occultist that some day the senses of hearing and sight will also be similarly distributed so that we shall both see and hear with our whole body and thus become still more sensitive in those respects than we are now.

Since then the pineal gland the pituitary body have become temporarily dormant (spiritually) to make man oblivious to the invisible world while he learns the lessons afforded by the material world. The pituitary body has manifested the Uranian influence sporadically in abnormal physical growth, producing freaks and monstrosities of various kinds, while Neptune working also abnormally through the pineal gland, has been responsible for the abnormal spiritual growth of medicine men, witches, and mediums of Spirit controls. When they are awakened to normal activities these two ductless glands will open the door to the inner worlds in a sane and safe manner, but in the meantime the thyroid gland, ruled by Mercury, the planet of reason, holds the secretion necessary to give the brain balance.

In the future the ductless glands are destined to play a prominent role; their development will accelerate evolution greatly, for their effects are mainly mental and spiritual. We are now nearing the Aquarian Age; the Sun is therefore beginning to transmit the highly intellectual vibrations of this sign which accounts for the intuitions, premonitions, and telepathic transmission now so prevalent. In the final analysis these phenomena are due to the awakening of the pituitary body, ruled by Uranus, the lord of Aquarius, and every passing year will make them more manifest.

THE LYMPHATIC SYSTEM:

The Lymphatic System is tubular and somewhat closely associated with the capillaries which connect the Venus and arterial circulations, terminating the large veins near the heart. The lymph which flows along its channel passes out one way, viz: toward the center of circulation, the heart. It is considered a system of small sewers for the body, simply because it collects the dish water of the tissues after they have all been bathed in the lymph which it carries. If you think of the tubes as drainage canals depleting the tissues of the wash water, you may think of these lymphatic glands as locks along the course of the channels at which the flow of lymph must stop and be filtered on its way to the Venus blood stream.

The glands are located in the bends of the elbows, in the arm pits, in the popliteal spaces, in the groins, thickly scattered throughout the anterior part of the neck (the part in front of the cervical vertebrae), in the abdomen between the folds of the mesentery which suspends the small intestines to the backbone, and in the chest between the lungs, this space being known as the mediastinum.

Every one of the lymphatic vessels passes through one or more of these glands on its way to its destination in the veins. The lymph cells are the only cells in the body that possess no cell wall; they move about like jellyfish in water. When inflammation attacks the human body in any of its types, the lymph is more responsible, for all poisonous liquids pass at once into the lymphatic channels.

The glands are likely to be sickly, owing to the poisonous nature of the lymph which filters through them. The lymphatic system is threefold: it collects lymph from the tissues, chyle from the intestines after it has been manufactured in the process of digestion, and by means of the lymphatic glands manufactures lymph cells which are identical with the white blood corpuscles.

CHAPTER II

THE VITAL BODY

EVOLUTION AND GENERAL PURPOSE:

The vital body is the second oldest of our vehicles, having its original germ given by the Lords of Wisdom in the Sun period. In the Sun Revolution of the Moon Period it was modified to render it capable of being interpenetrated by a desire body, also of accommodating itself to the nervous system, muscle, skeleton, etc.

During the Sun Revolution of the Earth Period the vital body was reconstructed to accommodate the germinal mind. It was fashioned at this time more in the likeness of the dense body, its organization at present being next to the dense body in efficiency.

Further reconstruction was done in the Hyperborean Epoch of the Earth Period when the Lords of Form appeared, with the Angels, and clothed man's dense form, then a baggy-shaped object, with a vital body.

The dense body is built into the matrix of the vital body during antenatal life, and with one exception, it is an exact copy, molecule for molecule, of the vital body. All through life the vital body is the builder and restorer of the dense form, its tendency being to soften, as well as to build. Its chief expression is the blood and the glands, also the sympathetic nervous system, having gained ingress into the stronghold of the desire body when it began to develop the heart into a voluntary muscle.

It interpenetrates the dense body and extends beyond its periphery about an inch and a half. In texture the vital body may be crudely compared to one of those picture frames made of hundreds of little pieces of wood which interlock and present innumerable points to the observer. The points of the vital body enter into the hollow centers of the dense atoms, imbuing them with vital force that sets them vibrating at a rate higher than that of the mineral of the Earth which is not thus accelerated and ensouled.

THE ETHERS AND THEIR FUNCTIONS:

When we analyze the human being, we find that in him all four ethers (the chemical, life, light and reflecting ethers) are dynamically active in the highly organized vital body. By means of the activities of the chemical ether he is able to assimilate food and to grow; the forces at work in the life ether enable him to propagate his species; the forces in the light ether supply the dense body with heat, work on the nervous system and the muscles, thus opening the doors of communication with the outside world by way of the senses; and the reflecting ether enables the Spirit to control its vehicles by means of thought. This ether also stores past experience as memory.

The chemical and life ethers form a matrix for our physical bodies. Each molecule of the physical body is embedded in a meshwork of ether which permeates and infuses it with life. Through these ethers the bodily functions, such as respiration, etc., are carried on, and the density and consistency of these matrices of ether determine the state of health.

The atoms of the chemical and life ethers gathered around the nuclear seed atom located in the solar plexus are shaped like prisms. They are all located in such a manner that when the solar energy enters our body through the spleen, the refracted ray is red. This is the color of the creative aspect of the Trinity, namely, Jehovah, the Holy Spirit, who rules Luna, the planet of fecundation. Therefore the vital fluid from the Sun which enters the human body by way of the spleen becomes tinged with a pale rose color, often noted by Seers when it courses along the nerves as electricity does in the wires of an electric system. Thus charged, the chemical and life ethers are the avenues of assimilation which preserve the individual, and of fecundation which perpetuates the race.

During life each prismatic vital atom penetrates a physical atom and vibrates it. To form a picture of this combination, imagine a pear-shaped wire basket having walls of spirally curved wire running obliquely from pole to pole. This is the physical atom; it is shaped nearly like our Earth, and the prismatic vital atom is inserted from the top, which is widest and corresponds to the north pole of our Earth. Thus the point of the prism penetrates the physical atom at the narrowest point, which corresponds to the south pole of the Earth, and the whole resembles a top swinging, swaying, and vibrating. In this manner our body is made alive and capable of motion.

The light and reflecting ethers are avenues of consciousness and memory. They are somewhat attenuated in the average individual and have not yet taken definite form; they interpenetrate the atom as air interpenetrates a sponge, and they form a slight auric atmosphere outside each atom.

It has been determined by physical science that the atoms in our dense body are constantly changing so that all the material which composes our present vehicle at this moment will have disappeared in a few years, but it is common knowledge that scars and other blemishes perpetuate themselves from childhood to old age. The reason for this is that the prismatic ether atoms which compose our vital body remain unchanged from the cradle to the grave. They are always in the same relative position--that is to say, the prismatic ether atoms which vibrate the physical atoms in the toes or in the fingers do not get to the hands, legs, or any other part of the body, but remain in exactly the same place where they were placed in the beginning. A lesion of the physical atoms involves a similar impression on the prismatic ether atoms. The new physical matter molded over them continues to take on shape and texture similar to those which originally obtained.

The foregoing remarks apply only to the prismatic atoms which correspond to solids and liquids in the Physical World, because they assume a certain definite shape which they preserve. But in addition each human being at this stage of evolution has a certain amount of light and reflecting ether, which are the vehicles of sense perception and memory, intermingled in his vital body. We may say that the light ether corresponds to the gases of our Physical World; perhaps the best description that can be given of the reflecting ether is to call it hyper-etheric. It is a vacuous substance of a bluish color resembling in appearance the blue core of a gas flame. It appears transparent and seems to reveal everything that is within it, but nevertheless it hides all the secrets of nature and humanity. In it is found one record of the memory of Nature. The light and reflecting ethers are of an exactly opposite nature to that of the stationary prismatic ether atoms. They are volatile and migratory. However much or little a man possesses of this material, it is an accretion, a fruitage, derived from his experiences in life. Inside the body it mingles with the blood stream and when it has grown by service and sacrifice in life's school so that it can no longer be contained within the body it is seen on the outside as a soul body of gold and blue.

Blue shows the highest type of spirituality, therefore it is smallest in volume and may be compared to the blue core of the gas flame, while the golden hue forms the larger part and corresponds to the yellow light which surrounds the core in the gas ring. The blue color does not appear outside the dense body save in the very greatest of saints--only yellow is usually observable there. At death this part of the vital body is etched into the desire body with the life panorama which it contains. The quintessence of all our life experience is then eventually impressed upon the seed atom as conscience or virtue which urges us to avoid evil and to do good in a coming life. Thus the quality of the seed atom is altered from life to life. The quintessence of good extracted from the migratory part of the vital body in one life determines the quality of the prismatic stationary ether atoms in the next life. The highest in one life becomes the lowest in the next and thus we gradually climb the ladder of evolution towards divinity.

From the foregoing it will be evident that the vital body is a vehicle of habit; all parents know that during the first seven years of childhood when this vehicle is in course of gestation that children form one habit after another. Repetition is the keynote of the vital body and habits depend upon repetition. It is different with the desire body, the vehicle of feelings and emotions which are always changing from moment to moment; though it has been said that the ether which forms our soul body is in constant motion and mingles with the blood stream, that motion is relatively slow compared to the rapidity of the current of the desire body; we may say that the ether moves like a snail compared with light.

When the Ego is on its way to rebirth through the Region of Concrete Thought, the Desire World, and the Etheric Region, it gathers a certain amount of material from each. The quality of this material is determined by the seed atom, on the principle that like attracts like. The quantity depends upon the amount of matter required by the archetype built by ourselves in the second Heaven. From the quantity of prismatic ether atoms that are appropriated by a certain Spirit, the Recording Angels and their agents build an etheric form which is then plead in the mother's womb and gradually clothed with physical matter which then forms the visible body of the new born child.

Only a small portion of the ether appropriated by a certain Ego is thus used, and the remainder of the child's vital body, or rather the material from which that vehicle will eventually be made, is thus outside the dense body. For that reason the vital body of a child protrudes much farther beyond the periphery of the dense body than does that of an adult. During the period of growth this store of ether atoms is drawn upon to vitalize the accretions within the body until, at the time when the adult age is reached, the vital body protrudes only from one to one and a half inches beyond the periphery of the dense body.

The Western Wisdom School teaches as its fundamental maxim that "all occult development begins with the vital body." The part of the vital body formed of the two higher ethers, the light ether and the reflecting ether, is what we may term the SOUL BODY; that is to say, it is more closely linked with the desire body and the mind and also more amenable to the Spirit's touch than are the two lower ethers. It is the vehicle of intellect, and responsible for all that makes man, man. Our observations, our aspirations, our character, etc., are due to the work of the Spirit in these two higher ethers, which become more or less luminous according to the nature of our character and habits. Also, as the dense body assimilates particles of food and thus gains in flesh, so the two higher ethers assimilate our good deeds during life and thus grow in volume as well. According to our doings in this present life we thus increase or decrease that which we brought with us at birth. This is the reason the Western Wisdom Teaching says that ALL MYSTIC DEVELOPMENT BEGINS WITH THE VITAL BODY.

CHAPTER III

THE DESIRE BODY AND THE MIND

In the third Revolution of the Moon Period the Lords of Individuality radiated from themselves the substance which they helped the unconscious, evolving man to appropriate and build into a germinal desire body. They also helped him to incorporate this germinal desire body in the compound vital body and dense body which he already possessed. This work was carried on all through the third and fourth Revolutions of the Moon Period.

The antagonistic "lower will" or will of the body, is an expression of the higher part of the desire body. When division of the Sun, Moon, and Earth took place, in the early part of the Lemurian Epoch, the more advanced portion of humanity-in-the-making experienced a division of the desire body into a higher and a lower part. The rest of humanity did likewise in the early part of the Atlantean Epoch.

This higher part of the desire body became a sort of animal soul. It build the cerebrospinal nervous system and the voluntary muscles, by that means controlling the lower part of the threefold body until the link of mind was given. Then the mind "coalesced" with the animal soul and became co-regent.

During the life of man his desire body is not shaped like his dense and vital bodies. After death it assumes that shape. During life it has the appearance of a luminous ovoid which, in waking hours, completely surrounds the dense body, as the albumen does the yolk of an egg. It extends from twelve to sixteen inches beyond the dense body in the ordinary individual. The matter in the human desire body is composed of material from the Desire World and is in incessant motion of inconceivable rapidity. There is in it no settled place for any particle, as in the dense body. The matter that is at the head one moment may be at the feet in the next and back again. There are no organs in the desire body, as in the dense and vital bodies, but there are centers of perception, which, when active, appear as vortices, always remaining in the same relative position to the dense body. In the majority of people they are mere eddies and are of no use as centers of perception. They may be awakened in all, however, but different methods produce different results. The desire body is rooted in the liver, and is born at about the fourteenth year in the being.

In the involuntary clairvoyant developed along improper, negative lines, these vortices turn from right to left, or in the opposite direction to the hands of a clock--counter-clockwise.

In the desire body of the properly trained voluntary clairvoyant, they turn in the same direction as the hands of a clock--clockwise, glowing with exceeding splendor, far surpassing the brilliant luminosity of the ordinary desire body. These centers furnish him with means for the perception of things in the Desire World and he sees, and investigates as he wills, while the person whose centers turn counter-clockwise is like a mirror, which reflects what passes before it.

In a far distant future man's desire body will become as definitely organized as are the vital and dense bodies. When that stage is reached we shall all have the power to function in the desire body as we now do in the dense body.

THE MIND:

In the Atlantean Epoch of the Earth Period the Lords of Mind radiated from themselves into our being the nucleus of material from which we are now seeking to build an organized mind. It was given to man to give purpose to action, but as the Ego was exceedingly weak and the desire nature strong, the nascent mind coalesced with the desire body; the faculty of Cunning resulted and was the cause of all the wickedness of the middle third of the Atlantean Epoch.

The mind, being the last of man's vehicles built, is not yet even a body. It is simply a link, a sheath for the use of the Ego as a focusing point. It is however, the most important instrument possessed by the Spirit, and its special instrument in the work of creation. We, ourselves, as Egos, function directly in the subtle substance of the Region of Abstract Thought, which we have specialized within the periphery of our individual aura. Thence we view the impressions made by the outer world upon the vital body through the senses, together with the feeling and emotions generated by them in the desire body, mirrored in the mind.

From these mental images we form our conclusions, in the substance of the Region of Abstract Thought, concerning the subjects with which they deal. These conclusions are ideas. By the power of will we project an idea through the mind, where it takes concrete shape as a thought form by drawing mind stuff around itself from the Region of Concrete Thought. The image may be projected in one of three directions:

(1) It may be projected against the desire body in an endeavor to arouse feeling which will lead to immediate action.

(2) Where no immediate action is called for by the mental images of impacts from without, these may be projected directly upon the reflecting ether, together with the thoughts occasioned by them, to be used at some future time.

(3) It may be projected toward another mind to act as a suggestion, to carry information, etc. When the work designed for such a thought form has been accomplished, or its energy expended in vain attempts to achieve its object, it gravitates back to its creator, bearing with it the indelible record of its journey.

At our present stage of evolution we say that the mind is born at the age of twenty-one, but the prime of mentality is not reached until about the forty-ninth year.

The mind is the focusing medium whereby the ideas wrought by the imagination of the Spirit are projected upon the material universe. First they are thought forms only, but when the desire to realize the imagined possibilities has set the man to work in the Physical World, they become what we call concrete "realities."

At the present time, however, the mind is not focused in a way that enables it to give a clear and true picture of what the Spirit imagines. It is not one-pointed. It gives misty and clouded pictures. Hence the necessity of experiment to show the inadequacies of the first conception, and bring about new imaginings and ideas until the image produced by the Spirit in mental substance has been reproduced in physical substance.

At the best, we are able to shape through the mind only such images as have to do with Form, because the human mind was not started until the Earth Period, and therefore is now in its form, or "mineral" stage, hence in our operations we are confined to forms, to minerals. We can imagine ways and means of working with the mineral forms of the three lower kingdoms, but can do little or nothing with living bodies. We may indeed graft living branch to living tree, or living part of animal or man to other living part, but it is not life with which we are working; it is form only. We are making different conditions, but the life which already inhabited the form continues to do so. To work with life is beyond man's power until his mind has become alive.

In the Jupiter Period the mind will be vivified to some extent and man can them imagine forms which will LIVE AND GROW, LIKE PLANTS.

In the Venus Period, when his mind has acquired "Feeling," he can create living, growing, and FEELING things.

When he reaches perfection, at the end of the Vulcan Period, he will be able to "imagine" into existence creatures that will live, grow, feel, and THINK.

CHAPTER IV

GENERAL CAUSES OF DISEASE

INTRODUCTION:

Disease is really a fire, the INVISIBLE FIRE which is THE FATHER endeavoring to break up the crystallized conditions which we have gathered in our bodies. We recognize fever as a fire, but tumors, cancers, and all other diseases are really also the effect of that invisible fire, which endeavors to purify the system and free it from conditions which we have brought about by breaking the laws of Nature.

Again, we may say that disease is a manifestation of ignorance, the only sin, and healing is a demonstration of applied knowledge, which is the only salvation. Christ is an embodiment of the Wisdom Principle, and in proportion as the Christ is formed in us we attain to health. Therefore, the healer should be spiritual and endeavor to imbue his patient with high ideals so that we may eventually learn to conform to God's laws which govern the universe, and thus attain permanent health in future lives as well as now.

The Old Testament opens with the account of how man was led astray by THE FALSE LIGHT of the Lucifer Spirits, giving birth to all the sorrow and suffering in the world; it closes with the promise that the Sun of Righteousness shall rise, with Healing in its wings. And in the New Testament we find the Sun of Righteousness, THE TRUE LIGHT, come to save world, and the first fact that is stated in regard to Him is that He is of Immaculate Conception.

Now this point should be thoroughly understood, that it is the Luciferian taint of passion which has brought sorrow, sin, and suffering into the world. When the creative power is used for sense gratification, whether in solitary or associated vice, with or without legal marriage, that is the sin which cannot be forgiven; it must be expiated. Humanity as a whole is now suffering for that sin.

The debilitated bodies, the sickness that we see around us has been caused by centuries of abuse, and until we learn to subdue our passions there can be no true health among the human race.

Prior to the impregnation of the desire body with this demoniac principle, conception was immaculate and a sacrament. Men walked in the presence of the Angels then, pure and unashamed. The act of fertilization was as chaste as that of the flower. Therefore when the mischief has been wrought, immediately the messenger, or Angel, girded them with leaves to impress upon them the ideal which they must learn to live, namely, that of the plant. Whenever we are able to perform the act of generation in a pure, chaste, and passionless manner as the plant does, an immaculate conception takes place and a Christ is born, capable of healing all the suffering of humanity, capable of conquering death and establishing immortality, a true light to lead humanity away from the will-o'-the-wisp of passion; through self-sacrifice to compassion.

This then is the great ideal toward which we are striving: to cleanse ourselves from the taint of egoism and self-seeking. Therefore we look upon the emblem of the Rose Cross as an ideal. The seven red roses typify the cleansed blood; the white rose shows the purity of life; and the golden radiating star symbolizes that inestimable influence for health, helpfulness and spiritual uplift which radiates from every SERVANT OF HUMANITY.

Until the Christ life illumines us from within we do not comprehend, neither do we follow, the laws of Nature, and consequently we contract diseases by our ignorant contravention of these laws. As Emerson put it, a man who is sick is a scoundrel in the act of being found out; he has broken the laws of Nature. That is why it is necessary that the gospel of Christ should be preached; that every one of us should learn to love our God with our whole heart and our whole soul and our brother as ourselves, for all our trouble in the world, whether we recognize it or not, comes from the one great fact of our selfishness. If the alimentative function is deranged, what is the reason? It is not that we have overtaxed our system because we have been angered, and exhausted our nervous force by trying to get someone to serve our selfish ends, and we feel resentful because we have not succeeded? In every case selfishness is the prime cause of most diseases; selfishness is the supreme besetting sin of ignorance.

CAUSES OF MENTAL DISABILITIES:

The disabilities which affect humanity may be divided into two large classes: MENTAL and PHYSICAL. The mental troubles are particularly traceable to the abuse of the creative function, when they are congenital, with one exception which we shall note later. The same holds true in case of impairment of the faculty of speech. This is reasonable and easy to understand. The brain and the larynx were built with half of the creative force by the Angels, so that man who, prior to the acquisition of these organs, was bisexual and able to create from himself alone, lost that faculty when these organs were created and is now dependent upon the cooperation of another of opposite polarity or sex in order to generate a new vehicle for an incoming Spirit.

When we use spiritual sight to look at man in the Memory of Nature during the time when he was yet in the making, we find that wherever there is now a nerve, there was first a desire current; that the brain itself was made of desire substance in the first place and also the larynx. It was desire that first sent a motive impulse through the brain and created these nerve currents, that the body might be moved and obtain for the Spirit whatever gratification was indicated by desire. Speech, also, is used for the purpose of obtaining a desired object or end. Through these faculties man has obtained a certain mastery over the world, and if he could just flit from one body to another, there would be no end to his abuse of his power for gratifying every whim and desire. But under the Law of Consequence he takes with him into a new body, faculties and organs similar to those which he left behind in the one preceding.

When passion has wrecked the body in one life, it is stamped upon the seed atom. In the next descent to rebirth it is therefore impossible for him to gather sound material with which to build a brain of stable construction. He is then usually born under one of the common signs, and usually also, the four common signs are on the angles; for through these signs passionate desire finds it difficult to express itself. Thus the powerful impulse which formerly ruled in his brain and which might be used for the purpose of rejuvenescence is absent; he lacks incentive in life and therefore he becomes helpless--a log upon the ocean of life--often insane.

But the Spirit is not insane; it sees, knows, and has a keen desire to use the body, though that may be an impossibility, for often it cannot even send a correct impulse along the nerves. The muscles of face and body are therefore not under the control of its will. This accounts for the lack of coordination which makes the maniac such a pitiable sight. And thus the Spirit learns one of the hardest lessons in life, namely, that it is worse than death to be tied to a living body and unable to find expression through it because THE DESIRE FORCE necessary to accomplish thought, speech, and motion HAS BEEN SPENT IN UNRIGHTEOUS LIVING in a previous life and left the Spirit without the necessary energy to operate its present fleshly instrument.

Though mental disabilities, when congenital, are generally traceable to abuse of the creative function in a past life, there is at least one notable exception to this rule: Where a Spirit, who has a particularly hard life before it, comes down to rebirth and feels upon entering the womb that the panorama of the coming life then shown it marks an existence too hard for it to undergo, it sometimes tries to run away from the school of life. At this time the Recording Angels or their agents have already made the connection between the vital body and the sense centers of the brain in the forming fetus; therefore the effort of the Spirit to escape from the mother's womb is frustrated, but the wrench that is given by the Ego deranges the connection between the etheric and physical sense centers, so that the vital body is not concentric with the physical, causing the etheric head to extend above the physical cranium. Thus it is impossible for the Spirit to use the dense vehicle; it is tied to a mindless body which it cannot use, and the embodiment is practically wasted.

We also find cases where a great shock later in life causes the Spirit to endeavor to run away with the invisible vehicles. As a result a similar wrench is given to the etheric sense centers in the brain, and the shock deranges the mental expression. Everybody has probably felt a similar sensation on receiving a fright; a surging as of something endeavoring to get out of the dense body; that is the desire and vital bodies, which are so swift in their action that an express train is as a snail by comparison. They see and feel the danger and are frightened before the scare is transmitted to the inert and slow physical body in which they are anchored, and which prevents their escape under ordinary strain.

But at times, as said, the fright and shock are sufficiently severe to give them such an impulse that the etheric sense centers are deranged. This most frequently happens to persons born under common signs, which are the weakest in the zodiac. However, as a ligament that has been stretched and torn may gradually regain comparative elasticity, so also, in these cases, it is easier to restore the mental faculties than in those cases where congenital insanity, brought over from past lives, has caused inadequate connection.

CAUSES OF PHYSICAL DISABILITIES:

With regard to physical abnormalities and deformities, the rule seems to be that as the physical indulgence of passion reacts on the mental state, so the abuse of the mental powers in one life leads to physical disability in later existences. An occult maxim says, "A lie is both murder and suicide in the Desire World." The teachings of the Elder Brothers given in THE ROSICRUCIAN COSMO-CONCEPTION explain that whenever an occurrence takes place, a certain thought form generated in the invisible world makes a record of the incident. Every time the event is talked about or commented upon, a new thought form is created which coalesces with the original and strengthens it, provided they are both true to the same vibration. But if an untruth is told concerning what happens, then the vibrations of the original and those of the reproduction are not identical; they jar and jangle, tearing each other to pieces. If the good and true thought form is sufficiently strong, it will overcome and break down the thought forms based upon a lie, and the good will overcome the evil but where the lies and malicious thoughts are the stronger, they may overcome the true thought form of the occurrence and thus demolish it. Afterwards they will jar among themselves, and all will in turn be annihilated. All things, in the ultimate, work together for good.

Thus a person who lives a clean life, endeavoring to obey the laws of God and striving earnestly for truth and righteousness, will create thought-forms about him of a corresponding nature; his mind will run in grooves that harmonize with truth; and when the time comes in the second heaven to create the archetype for his coming life, he will readily, intuitively, by force of habit from the past life, align himself with the forces of right and truth. These lines being built into his body, will create harmony in the coming vehicles, and health will therefore be his normal portion in the coming life. Those who, on the other hand, have in the past life taken a distorted view of things, displayed a disregard for truth, and exercised cunning, extreme selfishness, and a disregard for the welfare of others, are bound in the second heaven to see things in an oblique manner also, because that is their habitual line of thought. Therefore, the archetype built by them will embody lines of error and falsity; and consequently, when the body is brought to birth, it will exhibit a weakness in various organs, if not in the whole bodily organization.

Again we warn students not to draw quick conclusions from these tentative rules. It is not our intention to imply that everyone that has a seemingly healthy body has been a paragon of virtue in his past life, and he who suffers from one disability or another has been a scapegrace or good-for-nothing. None of us are able to tell at the present time "the whole truth and nothing but the truth." We are deceived because our senses are illusive. A long street seems to narrow in the distance, when, as a matter of fact, it is just as wide a mile away as where we are standing. The sun and the moon seem much larger when near the horizon than when at the zenith; but, as a matter of fact, we know that they do not gain in size by descending toward the horizon, nor lose by ascending into the mid-heaven. Thus we are constantly making allowances for and correcting sense illusions; similarly, with everything else in the world. What seems to be true is not always so, and what is true today regarding conditions of life may change tomorrow. Therefore it is impossible for us to know truth in the ultimate under the evanescent and illusory conditions of physical existence.

It is only when we enter the higher realms, and particularly into the Region of Concrete Thought, that the eternal verities are to be perceived; hence we must necessarily make mistakes again and again, even despite our most earnest efforts always to know and tell the truth. On that account it is impossible for us to build a thoroughly harmonious vehicle. Were that possible, such a body would really be immortal, and we know that immortality in the flesh is not the design of God. Paul says that "flesh and blood cannot inherit the kingdom of God."

But we know that even today only a very small percentage are ready to live as near the truth as they see it, to confess it and profess it before men by service and by righteous and harmless living. We can only understand that such must have been few and far between in the by-gone days, when man had not evolved the altruism that came to this planet with the advent of our Lord and Savior, Christ Jesus. The standards of morality were much lower then, and the love of truth almost negligible in the greater part of humanity, who were engrossed in their endeavors to accumulate as much wealth or gain as much power or prestige for themselves as possible. They were therefore naturally inclined to disregard the interests of others, and to tell a lie seemed in no way reprehensible and sometimes even appeared meritorious. The archetypes were constantly full of weaknesses, and the organic functions of the body today are interfered with to a serious degree as a result, particularly as the Western bodies are becoming more high strung and more sensitive to pain on account of the Spirit's growing consciousness.

CHAPTER V

SPECIFIC CAUSES OF DISEASE

INSANITY:

From the occultist's standpoint there are four classes of insanity. Insanity is always caused by a break in the chain of vehicles between the Ego and the physical body. This break may occur between the brain centers and the vital body, or it may be between the vital and desire body, between the desire body and the mind, or between the mind and the Ego. The rupture may be complete or only partial.

When the break is between the brain centers and the vital body, or between that and the desire body, we have the idiots. When the break is between the desire body and the mind, the violent and impulsive desire body rules and we have the raving maniac. When the break is between the Ego and the mind, the mind is the ruler over the other vehicles and we have the cunning maniac, who may deceive his keeper into believing that he is perfectly harmless until he has hatched some diabolical, cunning scheme. Then he may suddenly show his deranged mentality and cause a dreadful catastrophe.

There is one cause of insanity that it may be well to explain, as it is sometimes possible to avoid it. When the Ego is returning from the invisible world toward reembodiment, it is shown the various incarnations available. It sees the coming life in its great and general events, much as a moving picture passing before its vision. The it is given the choice, usually, of several lives. It sees at that time the lessons it has to learn, the fate it has generated for itself in past lives, and what part of that fate it will have to liquidate in each of the embodiments offered. The it makes its choice and is guided by the agents of the Recording Angels to the country and family where it is to live its coming life.

The panoramic view is seen in the Third Heaven where the Ego is naked and feels spiritually above sordid material considerations. It is much wiser then that is appears here on Earth, where it is blinded by the flesh to an inconceivable extent. Later, when conception has taken place and the Ego draws into the womb of its mother, on about the 18th day after that event, it comes in contact with the etheric mold of its new physical body which has been made by the Recording Angels to give the brain formation that will impress upon the Ego the tendencies necessary to work out its destiny.

There the Ego sees again the pictures of its COMING life as the drowning man perceives the pictures of his PAST life--in a flash. At that time the Ego is already partially blind to its spiritual nature, so that if the coming life seems to be a hard one, it will oftentimes shrink from entering the womb and making the proper brain connections. It may endeavor to draw itself out quickly and then, instead of being concentric as the vital and dense bodies should be, the vital body formed of ether may be drawn partially above the head of the dense body. In that case the connection between the sense centers of the vital body and the dense body are disrupted and the result is congenital idiocy, epilepsy, St. Vitus Dance, and similar nervous disorders.

The inharmonious relation between the parents which sometimes exists is often the last straw that makes an Ego feel that it cannot enter such an environment. Therefore, it cannot be too seriously impressed upon prospective parents that during the gestatory period it is of the utmost importance that every thing should be done to keep the mother in a condition of contentment and harmony. For it is a very hard task for the Ego to go through the womb; it taxes all its sensibilities to the very utmost, and inharmonious conditions in the home it is entering are, of course, an added source of discomfort, which may result in the above named dreadful state of affairs.

Black magic in its minor forms, such as hypnotism, for instance, sometimes causes congenital idiocy in a future life. The hypnotist deprives his victims of the free use of their bodies. Under the law of consequence he is then tied to a body with a malformed brain, which prevents his expression. We must not infer, however, that every case of congenital idiocy is due to such malpractice on the part of the Ego in a past life; there are also other causes which may bring congenital idiocy as a result.

Drugs and breathing exercises, such as the Eastern aspirant uses, have a dreadfully destructive effect upon the body, and it will therefore be seen that their use is altogether undesirable. Many a man is today in the insane asylum or in the grave of the consumptive on account of breathing exercises, and the effects of drugs are well known. The atoms of the Western body have been highly sensitized in the ordinary course of evolution, and the exercises which may be used with impunity by an Eastern person, whose body is not so highly sensitized, will cause the atoms of the Western body to run riot. It is extremely difficult to bring them into proper repose again.

MEDIUMSHIP:

Where a person becomes a medium for a disembodied Spirit which enters the body, as in the case of the trance medium where it takes possession of the body and uses it as the owner might do, there is little if any harm done, provided the Spirit control does not abuse his privilege. In fact, there are some cases where Spirit controls have better idea of caring for a body than the owner himself, and may sometimes improve the health. But Spirits of a high ethical nature do not usually control a medium, it is rather earthbound and low Spirits such as Indians and others of a like nature who obtain a control over mediumistic persons, and when in possession of the body they may use it to gratify their low passions for drink and sex. Thus they cause a disturbance to the system and a deterioration of the instrument.

In the case of the materializing medium, we may say that the influence is always injurious. The materializing Spirit entrances the victim and then draws the ether of the vital body out through the spleen, for the difference between the materializing medium and the ordinary person is the fact that the connection between the vital body and the dense body is exceedingly lax, so that it is possible to withdraw this vital body to a very great extent. The vital body is the vehicle whereby the solar currents which give us vitality are specialized. Deprived of the vitalizing principle, the body of the medium at the time of the materialization sometimes shrinks to almost one-half its usual size; the flesh becomes flabby and the spark of life burns very low. When the seance is over and the vital body replaced the medium is awakened and in normal consciousness. He then experiences a feeling of the most terrible exhaustion and sometimes, unfortunately, resorts to drink to revive the vital forces. In that case, of course, the health will very soon suffer and the medium will become a total wreck. At any rate, mediumship should be avoided, for apart from this danger to the instrument there are other and far more subtle bodies, and particularly in connection with the after-death state.

OBSESSION:

Obsession is a state where a discarnate Spirit has taken permanent possession of the body of someone after dispossessing the owner. But sometimes people who have formed the habit of drunkenness or some other low vice seek to excuse themselves by claiming to be obsessed. Wherever a person makes that statement concerning himself, one may nearly always be sure that it is nothing but an excuse, for a thief who has stolen something here in the material world does not go about and tell people of his theft, neither does an obsessing entity go around proclaiming the fact. It is very certain that such an entity does not care what is thought about the man whose body he has stolen, so that there is not reason why he should tell and risk being exorcised.

There is an infallible means of knowing whether a person is really obsessed, namely, by diagnosis of the eye. "The eye is the window of the soul," and only the true owner is capable of contracting and expanding the iris, or pupil of the eye, so that if we take a person who claims to be obsessed or whom we think is obsessed, to a room which is darkened, we shall find that the pupil of his eye will not expand if he is obsessed. Neither will the pupil contract when we bring him into the sunlight, nor expand if we ask him to look at an object at a distance or contract when he is asked to read small type. In short, the pupil of the eye will respond neither to light nor to distance when a person is obsessed, but there is also a certain disease called locomotor ataxia, where the iris will not respond to distance but is responsive to light.

No one who maintains a positive attitude of mind can ever become obsessed, for so long as we assert our individuality that is strong enough to keep all outsiders away. But in spiritualistic seances where the sitters are negative there is always a great danger. The best way to avoid becoming obsessed would be to maintain this positive attitude, and anyone who is at all negatively inclined should avoid going to spiritualistic seances, crystal gazing, and other methods of evoking spirits. This is bad practice, anyway, for those who have gone beyond have their work to do there and should not be brought back here.

At the moment of death when the seed atom in the heart, which contains all the experiences of the past life in a panoramic picture, is ruptured, the spirit leaves its physical body taking with it the finer bodies. It then hovers over the dense body which is now dead, as we call it, for a time varying from a number of hours to three and one-half days. The determining factor as to the time is the strength of the vital body, the vehicle which constitutes the soul body spoken of in the Bible. There is then a pictorial reproduction of the life, a panorama in reverse order from death to birth, and the pictures are etched upon the desire body through the medium of the reflecting ether in this vital body. During this time the consciousness of the Spirit is concentrated in the vital body, or at least it should be, and it has therefore no feeling about the matter. The picture that is impressed upon the vehicle of feeling and emotion, the desire body, is the basis of subsequent suffering in the life in Purgatory for evil deeds, and of enjoyment in the First Heaven on account of the good done in the past life.

The investigations of later years have revealed the additional fact that there is another process going on during these important days following death. A cleavage takes place in the vital body similar to that made by the process of initiation. So much of this vehicle as can be termed "soul," coalesces with the higher vehicles and is the basis of consciousness in the invisible worlds after death. The lower part which is discarded, returns to the physical body and hovers over the grave in the great majority of cases, as stated in the COSMO. This cleavage of the vital body is not the same in all persons but depends upon the nature of the life lived and the character of the person that is passing out. In extreme cases this division varies very much from normal. This important point was brought out in many cases of supposed spirit obsession which have been investigated from Headquarters; in fact it was these cases which developed the far-reaching and astounding discoveries brought out by our most recent researches into the nature of the obsession from which the people who appealed to us were suffering. As might be expected, of course, the division in these cases showed a preponderance of evil, and efforts were then made to find out if there were not also another class of people where a different division with a preponderance of good takes place. It is a pleasure to record that this was found to be the case, and after weighing the facts discovered, balancing one with another, the following seems to be a correct description of the conditions and their reasons:

The vital body aims to build the physical, whereas our desires and emotions tear down. It is the struggle between the vital body and the desire body which produces consciousness in the Physical World, and which hardens the tissues so that the soft body of the child gradually becomes tough and shrunken in old age, followed by death. The morality or immorality of our desires and emotions acts in a similar manner on the vital body. Where devotion to high ideals is the mainspring to action, where the devotional nature has been allowed for years to express itself freely and frequently, and particularly where this has been accomplished by the scientific exercises of Retrospection and Concentration, the quantity of the chemical and life ethers gradually diminishes as the animal appetites vanish, and an increased amount of the light and reflecting ether takes their place. As a consequence, the physical health is not as robust among people who follow the higher path as among people whose indulgence of the lower nature attracts the chemical and life ethers, in proportion to the extent and nature of their vice, to the partial or total exclusion of the two higher ethers.

Several very important consequences connected with death follow this fact. As it is the chemical ether which cements the molecules of the body in their places and keeps them there during life, when only a minimum of this material is present, disintegration of the physical vehicle after death must by very rapid. This the writer has not been able to verify because it is difficult to find men of high spiritual proclivities who have passed out recently, but it would seem that this is so from the fact recorded in the Bible that the body of Christ was not found in the tomb when the people came to look for it. As we have said before in relation to this matter, the Christ spiritualized the body of Jesus so highly, made it so vibrant, that it was almost impossible to keep the particles in place during His ministry. As stated before, a worldly life increases the proportion of the lower ethers in the vital body to that of the higher. Where, in addition, a so-called "clean life" is lived and excesses avoided, the health during life is more robust than that of the aspirant to the higher life, because the latter's attitude to life builds a vital body composed principally of the higher ethers. He loves "the bread of life" more than physical sustenance and therefore his instrument becomes increasingly high-strung, nervous, and delicate, a sensitive conditions which greatly furthers the objects of the Spirit, but which is a hardship from the physical viewpoint.

In the majority of mankind there is such a preponderance of selfishness and a desire to get the most out of life as they view that matter, that either they are busy keeping the wolf from the door or accumulating possessions and taking care of them, and hence they have very little time or inclination to undertake the soul culture so necessary to true success in life.

Therefore there is so little that persists in each life of the majority and evolution is so frightfully slow that until one is able to view the act of death from the higher regions of the World of Concrete Thought and, so to say, look downwards, it does not appear that anything is saved of the vital body. This body seems to return complete to the physical body and hover over the grave, there to disintegrate simultaneously with the latter. As a matter of fact, an increasing part cleaves to the higher vehicles and goes with them into the desire world, there to be a basis of consciousness in, and to live through, the purgatorial and heaven lives, generally persisting until man enters the second heaven and unites with the nature forces there in his efforts to create for himself a new environment. By that time, it has been absorbed by the spirit or almost so, and whatever may remain of a material nature will quickly fade away.

But there are some people who are of such an evil nature that they ENJOY a life spent in vice and degenerate practices, a brutal life, and who delight in giving pain. Sometimes they even cultivate the occult arts for evil purposes so that they may have a greater power over their victims. Then their fiendish, immoral practices result in hardening their vital body.

In such extreme cases where the animal nature has been paramount, where there has been no soul expression in the preceding Earth life, the division in the vital body spoken of before cannot take place at death, for there is no dividing line. In such a case, if the vital body should gravitate back to the dense body and there gradually disintegrate, the effect of a very evil life would not be so far-reaching, but unfortunately there is in such cases an interlocking grip of the vital and the desire bodies which prevents separation. We have seen that where a man lives mostly in the higher nature, his spiritual vehicles are nourished to the detriment of the lower. Conversely, where his consciousness is centered in the lower vehicles, he strengthens them immeasurably. It should be understood that the life of the desire body is not terminated by the departure of the spirit; it has a residual life and consciousness. The vital body is also able to sense things in a slight measure for a few days after death in ordinary cases (hence the suffering caused by embalming, post-mortem examinations, etc., immediately after death), but where a low life has hardened and endured it with great strength, it has a tenacious hold on life and an ability to feed on odors of foods and liquors. Sometimes, as a parasite, it even vampirizes people with whom it comes in contact.

Thus an evil man may live for many, many years unseen in our very midst, yet so close that he is nearer than hands and feet. He is far more dangerous than the physical criminal for he is able to prompt others of a similar bent to criminal or degenerate practices without fear of detection or punishment by law.

Such beings are therefore one of the greatest menaces to society imaginable. They have sent countless victims to prison, broken up homes and caused an unbelievable amount of unhappiness. They always leave their victims when the latter have come into the clutches of the law. They gloat over their victim's sorrow and distress, this being a part of their fiendish scheme. It is amazing when one searches the Memory of Nature of the past to find how prevalent this interlocking condition of the desire and vital bodies was in former centuries and millenniums. We realize, of course, in a sort of an abstract way, that the farther we go back into the history of men the more savage we find them, but that in our own historical times this savagery should have been so common and so brutal and that might was the measure of right absolutely and beyond dispute, was, to say the least, quite a shock to the writer. It has been taught that selfishness and desire were purposely fostered under the regime of Jehovah to give incentive to action. This in the course of time had so hardened the desire body that when the advent of Christ took place, there was almost no heaven life among the people then living.

Earthbound Spirits, such as previously mentioned, gravitate to the lower regions of the Desire World which interpenetrates the ether, and are in constant and close touch with those people on

Earth most favorably situated for aiding them in their evil designs. They usually stay in the earthbound condition for fifty, sixty, or seventy-five years, but extreme cases have been found in which such people so remain for centuries.

When the Spirit has left the SIN BODY, as we call this body in contrast to the soul body, to ascend to the Second Heaven, it does not disintegrate as quickly as the ordinary shell left behind by normal people, for the consciousness in it is enhanced by its dual composition; that is to say, being composed of both a vital and desire body, it has an individual or a personal consciousness that is very remarkable. It cannot reason, but there is a low cunning present which makes it seem as though it were actually endowed with a spiritual presence, an Ego, and this enables it to live a separate life for many centuries. The departed Spirit meanwhile enters the Second heaven, but having done no work on Earth to desire or merit a prolonged stay there or in the Third heaven, it only stays there sufficiently long to create a new environment for itself and it is then reborn much earlier than usual--to satisfy the cravings for material things which draw it so strongly.

When the Spirit returns to Earth, this sin body is naturally attracted towards it, and usually stays with it all its life as a demon. Investigations have proved that this class of soulless creatures were very prevalent during Biblical times, and it was to them that our Savior referred as devils, they being the cause of various obsessions and bodily ills such as are recorded in the Bible.

In addition to the entities already mentioned who dwell in a sin body made by themselves, and who thus suffer entirely from their own deeds in the period of expiation, two classes were found which were similar in certain respects although different in others. In addition to the divine Hierarchies and the four life waves of Spirits now evolving in the Physical World through the mineral, plant, animal, and human kingdoms, there also other life waves which express themselves in the various invisible worlds. Among them there are certain classes of sub-human spirits which are called elementals. It sometimes happens that one of these elementals takes possession of the sin body of some one of a savage tribe, and thus adds extra intelligence to that being. At the rebirth of the spirit that generated this sin body, the usual attracting brings them together, but on account of the elemental ensouling the sin body, the spirit becomes different from the other members of the tribe, and we find them then acting as medicine men or in a similar capacity. These elemental spirits ensouling the sin bodies of Indians also act upon mediums as spirit controls, and having obtained power over the medium during life, when he dies, these elemental controls oust him from the vehicles which contain his life experience. Thus the medium may be retarded in evolution for ages, for there is no power that can compel these spirits to let go, once they have gained control of such a body. Therefore, though mediumship may produce no seeming evil effect in a lifetime, there is a very, very grave danger after death to the person who allows another to take possession of his body.

HYSTERIA, EPILEPSY, TUBERCULOSIS, AND CANCER:

Hysteria, epilepsy, tuberculosis, and cancer were all found to result from the erratic propensities of a past life. It was noticed that though many of the subjects had been, in the past lives investigated, almost maniacal in the gratification of their lasciviousness, they were at the same that the physical body generated in the present life was normally healthy and their disability altogether mental, while in other cases where the indulgence of the passional nature was coupled with a vile character and a cruel disregard of others, epilepsy together with rachitis, hysteria, and a deformed body were the present result. Frequently, cancer, especially cancer of the liver or breast resulted.

In this connection, however, we wish again to warn students not to draw hasty conclusions that these are hard and fast conditions. The number of investigations made, though very large and an arduous task for one researcher to handle, are too few to be really conclusive in matters involving millions of human beings. They are, however, in line with the teachings of the COSMO given by the Elder Brothers regarding the effect of materialism in bring about rachitis, a softening of a part of the body that should be hard, and tuberculosis, which hardens tissues that should be soft and pliable. Cancer is essentially similar in effect; and when we consider that the sign Cancer is ruled by the Moon, the planet of generation, and that the lunar sphere is under the sway of Jehovah, the God of generation, whose Angels announce and preside over birth as instanced in the case of Isaac, Samuel, John the Baptist, and Jesus, we readily see that abuse of the creative function can cause both cancer and lunacy in the most differentiated forms.

IMPAIRMENT OF VISION:

Regarding lack of vision or disabilities or the organ of sight, it has long been known among researches that it is the effect of extreme cruelty in a past life. Recent investigations have developed the further information that much of the eye trouble now prevalent among people is due to the fact that OUR EYES ARE CHANGING; they are, in fact, becoming responsive to a higher octave of vision that before, because the ether surrounding the Earth is becoming more dense and the air is growing more rarer. This is particularly true in certain parts of the world, Southern California among others. It is noteworthy in this connection that the Aurora Borealis is becoming more frequent and more powerful in its effects upon the Earth. In the early years of the Christian Era this phenomenon was almost unknown, but in the course of time as the Christ wave which descends into the Earth during part of the year, infuses more and more of its own life into the dead, earthly lump, the ETHERIC VITAL RAYS become visible at intervals. Later they became more and more numerous and are now commencing to interfere with our electric activities, particularly with telegraphy, which service is sometimes completely demoralized by these radiating streamers.

It is also noteworthy that the disturbances are confined to wires going east and west. Rays or lines of force from the plant Group Spirits, radiate in all directions from the center of the Earth towards the periphery and then outwards, passing through the roots of plants or trees, then upwards towards the top of same.

The currents of the animal Group Spirits, on the other hand, encircle the Earth. The comparatively weak and invisible currents generated by the Group Spirits of the plants, and the very strong powerful rays of force generated by the Christ Spirit now becoming visible as the Aurora Borealis, have hitherto been of about the same nature as static electricity, while the currents generated by the animal Group Spirits and which encircle the Earth may be likened to dynamic electricity which gave the Earth its power of motion in bygone ages. Now, however, the Christ currents are becoming more and more forceful and their static electricity is being liberated. The etheric impulse which they give will inaugurate a new era, and the sense organs now possessed by mankind must accommodate themselves to this change. Instead of the etheric rays which emanate from an object bringing a reflected image to the retina of our eyes, the so-called "blind spot" will be sensitized and we shall look out through the eye and see directly the thing itself instead of the image upon our retina. Then we shall not only see the surface of the thing we observe, but we shall be able to see through it as those who have cultivated the etheric vision do now.

As time goes on and the Christ by His beneficent ministration attracts more and more of the interplanetary ether to the Earth, thus making its vital body more luminous, we shall be walking in a sea of light, and when we learn to forsake our ways of selfishness and egotism through the constant contact with these beneficent Christ vibrations, we shall also become luminous. Then the eye as it is now constituted would not be of service to is, therefore it is now beginning to change and we are experiencing the discomfort incident to all reconstruction.

SHELL SHOCK:

It was found by examining a number of people in normal health that each of the prismatic atoms composing the lower ethers radiated from itself the lines of force which set spinning the physical atom in which it is inserted, enduring the whole body with life. The united trend of all these units of force is toward the periphery of the body, where they constitute what has been called the "Odic Fluid," also designated by other names. When the air pressure from without is lowered by residence in a high altitude, a tendency to nervousness becomes manifest because the etheric force from within rushes outward unchecked; and were the man not able to shut off the outflow of solar energy in part by an effort of will to overcome the difficulty, no one could live in such a place.

We have heard of "shell shock" and we are aware that numbers of people who had not even the slightest wound were found dead on the battlefield. In fact, we had seen and spoken with people who had passed out in this manner but were at a loss to know why death had resulted. They all disclaimed fear and were unanimous in their assertion that they had suddenly become unconscious and a moment later they had found themselves in their present condition. They were unlike their fellows in that they had not a single scratch on their bodies. Our preconceived idea that it must have been a momentary fear at a particularly close call which, though unrealized, had caused their demise, prevented a full investigation; but the ascertained results of the consequences of a fall led us to believe that something similar might take place in this connection; this surmise was correct.

One night some time ago while in transit to a place in a far country where I had a mission to perform, I heard a cry. Though the human voice can be heard only in air, there are overtones which are heard in the spiritual realms at distances exceeding those traversed by wireless messages. The cry was close by, however, and I was on the scene in an instant, but not soon enough to give the needed help. I found a man sliding down a slanting embankment, bare of vegetation, perhaps a dozen feet in width, and as it proved on subsequent examination, almost smooth, and without a fissure which would have afforded a hold for his fingers. To have saved him would have involved materialization of both hands and shoulders, but there was no time. In a moment he had slid over the overhanging precipice and was falling to the floor of the canyon below, probably several thousand feet.

Prompted by a natural spirit of fellow feeling I followed and on the way observed the phenomenon which is the way observed the phenomenon which is the basis of this article, namely, that when the body had attained a considerable velocity, the ethers composing the vital body commenced to ooze out, and when the body crashed to rocks below, a mangled mass, there was very little if any ether left in it. Gradually, however, the ethers drifted together, took form, and hovered with the finer vehicles above the mangled corpse; but the man was in a stupor and unable to sense or realize the fact of his altered condition.

As soon as I saw that he was beyond help, I went on; but on thinking the matter over it dawned on me that something unusual had happened and that it was my duty to find out if the ethers left that way in everyone who fell, and if so, why. Under old time conditions this would have been difficult, but the advent of the flying machine claims many victims. It was therefore easy to ascertain the fact that when a falling body has attained a certain velocity, the higher ethers leave the dense body, and the falling man becomes insensible. As the body reaches the ground, it is mangled, but the poor man may regain consciousness when the ether has reorganized itself. He will then begin to suffer from the physical consequences of the fall. If the fall continues after the higher ethers have left, the increased velocity dislodges the lower ethers, and the silver cord is all that remains attached to the body. This is ruptured at the moment of impact with the ground, and the seed atom passes on to the breaking point, where it is held in the usual way.

From these facts we came to the conclusion that is the normal air pressure which holds the vital body within the dense. When we move with an abnormal velocity, the pressure is removed from some parts of the body and a partial vacuum formed, with the further result that the ethers leave the body and flow into this vacuum. The two higher ethers, which are most loosely bound, are the first to disappear and leave the man senseless after they have produced the panorama of life in a flash. Then if the fall continues to increase the air pressure in front of the body and the vacuum behind, the more closely bound lower ethers are also forced out, and the body is dead before it reaches the ground.

When a large projective passes through the air, it creates a vacuum behind it by the enormous velocity wherewith it moves, and if the person is within this vacuum zone while the shell is passing, he suffers in a measure determined by his own nature and his proximity to the center of suction. His position is in fact a reverse replica of the man who falls; for he stands still while a moving body removes the air pressure and allows the ethers to escape. If the amount of ether dislocated is comparatively slight and is composed only of the third and fourth ethers which govern sense perception and memory, he will probably suffer only a temporary loss of memory and inability to sense things or move. This disability will disappear when the extracted ethers are again fitted inside the dense body--a much more difficult achievement than where the physical body succumbs and the reorganization takes place without reference to that vehicle.

SCLEROSIS OR HARDENING OF THE ARTERIES:

Our bodies are gradually hardening from childhood to old age, on account of the chalky substances contained in most of the foods we usually nourish our bodies upon. This calcareous matter is primarily deposited in the walls of the arteries and veins, causing what is known to the medical profession as arterio-sclerosis or hardening of the arteries. The arteries of a little child are exceedingly soft an elastic, like a rubber tube, but gradually as we advance through childhood, youth, and on toward old age, the walls of the arteries become harder in consequence of the deposits of chalk left by the passing blood. Thus in time they may become as stiff and inelastic as a pipe stem. There is a condition which is called pipe-stem artery. The arteries then become brittle and may break, causing hemorrhage and death. Therefore it is truly said that a man is as old as his arteries. If we can clear the arteries and capillaries of this earthy matter, we may gradually prolong life and the usefulness of our body.

From the occult standpoint, of course, it is no matter whether we live or die, as the saying is, for death to us does not mean annihilation but only the shifting of the consciousness to other spheres; nevertheless, when we have brought a vehicle through the useless years of childhood past the hot years of youth, and have come to the time of discretion when we are really beginning to gain experience, then the longer we can prolong the time of experience the more we may gain. For that reason it is of a certain value to prolong the life of the body.

In order to accomplish that result, we must first select the foods that are least impregnated with the choking substances which cause the induration of arteries and capillaries. These may be briefly stated to be the green vegetables and all fruits. next, it is of importance to seek to eradicate the choking matter which we have already absorbed, if that is possible, but science has not yet found any food or medicine that will with certainty produce that effect. Electric baths have been found to be exceedingly beneficial but not entirely satisfactory. Buttermilk is the best agent for eradicating this earthy substance and next comes grape juice. If taken continually and in generous quantities, these substances will considerably ameliorate the hardened condition of the arteries.

CHAPTER VI

HEREDITY AND DISEASE

Unfortunately, people seem to lay their bad traits to heredity, blaming their parents for their faults, while taking to themselves all the credit for the good. The very fact that we differentiate between that which is inherited and that which is our own shows that there are two sides to man's nature, the side of the FORM, and the life side.

We are drawn to certain people by the law of causation, and the law of association. The same law which causes musicians to seek the company of one another in concert halls, gamblers to congregate at the race tracks or in pool rooms, people of a studious nature to flock to libraries, etc., also causes people of similar tendencies, characteristics, and tastes to be born in the same family. When we hear a person say, "Oh, yes, I know I am extravagant, but I just cannot help it. It runs in the family," it is the law of association; and the sooner we recognize, that instead of making the law of heredity an excuse for our evil habits, we should seek to conquer them and cultivate virtues instead, the better for us.

Man is essentially spirit and he comes here equipped with a mental and moral nature, which are entirely his own, taking from his parents only the material for the physical body. Thus while heredity in the first place is true only as regards the material of the dense body and not the soul qualities, which are entirely individual, the incoming Ego also does a certain amount of work on its dense body, incorporating in it the quintessence of its past physical qualities. No body is an exact mixture of the qualities of its parents, although the Ego is restricted to the use of the materials taken from the bodies of the father and mother. Hence a musician incarnates where he can get the material to build the slender hand and the delicate ear, with its sensitive fibres of Corti and its accurate adjustment of the three semicircular canals. The arrangement of these materials, however, is to the extent named, under the control of the Ego.

In the fetus, in the lower part of the throat just above the sternum or breast bone, there is a gland called the thymus gland, which is largest during the period of gestation and which gradually atrophies as the child grows older and disappears entirely by or before the fourteenth year, very often when the bones have been properly formed. Science has been very much puzzled as to the use of this gland, and few theories have been advanced to account for it. Among these theories one is that it supplies the material for the manufacture of the red blood corpuscles until the bones have been properly formed in the child so that it may manufacture its own blood corpuscles. That theory is correct.

During the earliest years the Ego which owns the child-body is not in full possession, and we recognize that the child is not responsible for its doings, at any rate not before the seventh year, and later we have extended it to the fourteenth year. During that time no legal liability for its action attaches to the child, and that it as it should be, for the Ego being in the blood can only function properly in blood of its own making, so that where, as in the child-body, the stock of the blood is furnished by the parents through the thymus gland, the child is not yet its own master or mistress. Thus it is that children do not speak of themselves so much as "I" in the earlier years, but identify themselves with the family; they are Papa's girl and Mama's boy. The young child will say "Mary wants this" or "Johnny wants that," but as soon as they have attained the age of puberty and have begun to manufacture their own blood corpuscles, then we hear the boy or girl say, "I" will do this or "I" will do that. From that time they begin to assert their own identify, and to tear themselves loose from the family.

Seeing, then, that the blood throughout the years of childhood, as well as the body, is inherited from the parents, the tendencies to disease are also carried over, not the disease itself, but the tendency. After the fourteenth year, when the indwelling Ego has commenced to manufacture its own blood corpuscles, it depends a great deal upon itself whether or not these tendencies shall become manifested actualities in its life.

CHAPTER VII

EFFECTS OF ALCOHOL AND TOBACCO

Flesh and alcohol have the tendency to make man ferocious and to turn his spiritual sight away from the higher worlds and focus vision upon the present material plane. Therefore the Bible tells us that at the beginning of the rainbow age, the age where we live in an atmosphere of clear and pure air, so different from the misty atmospheric condition of Atlantis spoken of in the second chapter of Genesis, Noah first brewed wine. Material development has taken place in consequence of the present focusing of our energies upon the material world, which resulted from partaking of meat and wine.

Christ's first miracle changed water into wine. HE HAD RECEIVED THE UNIVERSAL SPIRIT at the baptism, and had no need of artificial stimulants. He changed the water to wine to give to others less advanced. But no wine bibbers can inherit the kingdom of God. The esoteric reason is this, that while the lower ethers vibrate to the seed atoms in the solar plexus and the heart, and thus keep the physical body alive, the higher ethers vibrate to the pituitary body and pineal gland. By imbibing this false rebellious spirit that is fermented OUTSIDE the body, and is different from the spirit that is fermented INSIDE, by sugar, these organs are temporarily dazed and cannot vibrate to the higher world, and so because of age-long abuse, man has ceased to function in the higher worlds. If he takes too much of this spirit of alcohol, the organs named may be slightly awakened so that he sees the lowest realms of the desire world and all the evil things therein; that happens in the disease known as delirium tremens. To sum up, as the evolution of soul depends upon acquisition of the two higher ethers from which the beautiful wedding garment is made, and as these ethers are attuned to the organs named in the same manner that the lower ethers are attuned to the seed atom in the heart and the seed atom in the solar plexus, you will readily understand the deadly effects to the spiritual man, of alcohol and drugs. To elucidate further I quote an incident of life.

There is an old saying: "Once a Mason always a Mason"; that means that when anyone has received the initiation of the Masonic Order, and by virtue of that becomes a Mason, he cannot resign, for he cannot give up that knowledge and the secrets which he has learned any more than a person who goes to college can give back his learning received at that institution and therefore, once a Mason always a Mason, and likewise, once a pupil, a lay brother, of a mystery school, always a pupil and a lay brother of said same mystery school. But though that holds good and life after life we come back connected with the same order that we have been affiliated with in previous lives, we may in any one life so conduct ourselves that it is impossible for us to realize this in our physical brains, and I will, as said, cite for the benefit of all students a case which is very much to the point.

When I was taken into the Temple of the Rosicrucian order in Germany I was surprised to see a man whom I had known on the Pacific Coast; that is to say I had seen him a few times; we had never spoken. He seemed at that time to be in a station in the society, where we were connected, much above mine, and I had never had personal acquaintance with him. However, he greeted me there warmly, and seemed to understand all about his connection with said society, about our meeting there, and so forth; and I looked forward upon my return to America to getting much information from this brother when I should be fortunate enough to meet him here in the West. When I arrived at the city where he was, I was told by mutual friends that he had been expecting me and was looking forward anxiously to meeting me. Therefore, when I did meet the gentleman, I at once went up to him and shook him by the hand. He also seemed to recognize me and called me by name. It seemed there was every indication that he knew all that had happened while we were both out of the body. Besides, he had told me in the Temple that he remembered everything that happened to him when out of the body; this of course I believed for he was of a much higher degree than the first, into which I had just been admitted.

On the day of our physical meeting, after a few moments' conversation I said something which caused him to stare at me blankly. I had referred to some incident of our meeting in the Temple, and he showed plainly that he knew nothing whatever of it. I had, however, said so much that I was forced to say more, or appear very foolish so I told him that he had professed to remember everything. This he denied, and at the end of the interview he begged me very earnestly to endeavor to find out why it was that he was a lay brother of the Rosicrucian Order, yet could not remember that which took place during his absence from the body. He was as I knew at various Temple services. He took part, yet in his physical brain he was absolutely ignorant of that which had occurred. The mystery was solved a little later when I learned from him, out of the body, the fact that he smoked cigarettes and used drugs which clouded his brain to such an extent that it had become impossible for him to carry anything through of his psychic experiences. When I told him that in the body, he made a valiant effort to rid himself of the habit which he acknowledged. This case illustrates how careful we should be to be clean in our habits; in everything to regard this body of ours as the Temple of God, and refrain from defiling it as we would refrain from defiling a house of God built of stone and mortar, which is not one millionth part as holy as the body wherewith we have been endowed. The brain, in particular, is the great and important instrument whereby we are doing our work in the Physical World, and we obviously should not use any intoxicants or drugs which muddle it and thus prevent our making the progress we expect.

CHAPTER VIII

ORIGIN AND DEVELOPMENT OF HEALING

It is a trite saying that "man if of few days and full of trouble." Among all the vicissitudes of life none affects us more powerfully than loss of health. We may lose fortunes or friends with comparative equanimity, but when health fails and death threatens, the strongest falter; realizing human impotence we are more ready to turn to divine power for succor then than at other times. Therefore, the office of spiritual adviser has always been closely associated with healing.

Among savages the priest was also "medicine man." In ancient Greece, Aesculapius was particularly sought by those in need of healing. The church followed in his steps. Certain Catholic orders have continued the endeavor to assuage pain during the centuries which have intervened between that day and the resent. In times of sickness the "good Father" came as a representative of our Father in Heaven, and what he lacked in skill was made up by love and sympathy--if he was indeed a true and holy priest--and by the faith engendered in the patient by the priestly office. His care of the patient did not commence at the sick bed, nor was it terminated at recovery. The gratitude of the patient toward the physician was added to the veneration felt for the spiritual adviser, and as a consequence the power of the priest to help and uplift his erstwhile patient was enormously increased, and the tie between them was closer than possible where the offices of spiritual and medical adviser are divorced.

It is patent that the art of medicine has reached a stage of efficiency which could not have been attained save by devotion to that one particular end and aim. The safeguards of sanitary laws, the extinction of insect carriers of disease are monumental testimonies to the value of modern scientific methods. Thus it may seem as if all were well and there were no need of further effort. But in reality, until humanity as a whole enjoys perfect health, there is no issue more important than the question, How may we attain and maintain perfect health?

In addition to the regular school of surgery and medicine, which depends exclusively upon physical means for the care of disease, other systems have sprung up which depend entirely on mental healing. It is the custom of organizations which advocate "mind cure," "nature cure," and other like methods to hold experience meetings and publish journals with testimonials from grateful supporters who have benefited by their treatments, and if physicians of the regular school did likewise there would be no lack of similar testimonies of their efficiency.

The opinion of thousands is of great value, but it does not prove anything, for thousands may hold an opposite view. Occasionally a single man may be right and the rest of the world wrong, as when Galileo maintained that the Earth moves. Today the whole world has been converted to the opinion for which he was persecuted as a heretic. We maintain that as man is a composite being, cures are successful in proportion as they remedy defects on the physical, moral, and mental planes of being.

CURING VS. HEALING:

As the great majority of people do not make a distinction between curing and healing, it may be well to explain the difference which is primarily one of cooperation or the lack thereof. One person may undertake to "cure" another by massage or drugs; the patient in either of these cases is passive as the clay that is being molded by the potter. There is no doubt that under such treatment trouble may disappear and the person be made well, but this is only a temporary relief: he has not received the proper appreciation of the underlying cause of his disease, he does not understand that the illness was a consequence of breaking the laws of Nature, and is therefore very liable to go and do the same things over again with the result that his malady returns. A "cure" is a physical process. Healing is radically different; there the sufferer is always required to cooperate both spiritually and physically with the healer.

To make this clear we can do not better than view the life and work of our great Leader, the Christ. When people came to Him to be healed they did not expect a physical treatment, but knew that relief would be given through the power of the Spirit. They had unlimited confidence in Him, and that this was essential we see from the incidents recorded in the thirteenth chapter of Matthew where He is said to have gone among the people with whom Jesus, the original owner of the body, had dwelt in early youth. They saw only the outward man: "Is this not Jesus, the son of Joseph; are not his brethren with us?" etc. They believed that nothing great could come out of Nazareth, and according to their faith it was done unto them, for we read that "He did not many mighty works there because of their unbelief."

But faith without works is dead, and in every case where Christ healed anyone, this person had to do something; he had to cooperate actively with the great Healer before his cure could be accomplished. He said, "Stretch forth thy hand," and when the man did so the hand was healed; to another, "Take up thy bed and walk," and when he did so the malady disappeared; to the blind, "Go and bathe in the pool of Siloam"; to the leper, "Show thyself to the priest, offer your gifts," etc. In every case there was active cooperation upon the part of the one to be healed, which helped the Healer. They were simple requirements, but such as they were they had to be complied with, so that the spirit of obedience could aid the Healer's work. When Naaman came to Elijah and thought that this prophet was going to come out with a great show of magic and ceremony to dispel the leprous spots from his body he was domed to disappointment. And when the prophet sent word to him, "Go and wash seven times in the river Jordan," he was enraged to the point of crying out, "Have we not great rivers in Assyria and why should I go and wash in the Jordan? What nonsense!" He lacked the spirit of submission which is absolutely necessary in order that the work may be done, and it is safe to say that had he persisted he would not have received the healing of his malady. Neither would any of those who were healed by his malady. Neither would any of those who were healed by the Christ have been affected unless they had obeyed and had done as they were bidden. This is a law of Nature that is absolutely sure. It is disobedience that brings disease. Obedience, no matter whether that involves washing in the Jordan or stretching forth a hand, shows a change of mind, and the man is therefore in a position to receive the healing balm which may come through the Christ, or through a healer of one kind or another as the case may be. Primarily, in all cases, the healing force comes our Heavenly Father, Who is the Great Physician.

These are the three great factors in healing: first, the power, from our Father in Heaven; next, the healer, and third, the obedient mind of the patient upon which the power of the Father can act through the healer in such a way as to dispel all bodily ills.

Let us now understand that the whole universe is pervaded with the power of the Father, always available to cure all ills of whatever nature; that is the great certainty.

The healer is the focus, the vehicle through which the power is infused into the patient's body. If he is a proper instrument, consecrated, harmonious, really and truly in tune with the Infinite, there is no limit to the wonderful works of the Father which may be performed through him when opportunity presents a patient of a properly receptive and obedient mind.

CHAPTER IX

THE ROSICRUCIAN FELLOWSHIP METHOD OF HEALING

WHY THE ROSICRUCIANS HEAL:

Among all the foolish and fallacious nonsense which has been circulated concerning the Rosicrucians during the past centuries, there is one great truth: "Members of the Order aim to heal the sick and have superior means of accomplishing this benevolent purpose." Earlier religious orders have sought to advance spiritually by castigating and abusing the body, but the ROSICRUCIANS exhibit the tenderest care for this instrument. There are two reasons for their healing activities. Like all other earnest followers of Christ they are longingly looking for "the day of the Lord." They know that Lucifer, the false Light of Lemuria, implanted passion, inaugurating BEGETTAL IN SIN, and caused sorrow, pain and death; also that Christ, the true Light of the coming New Galilee, inaugurated the IMMACULATE CONCEPTION, and preached the gospel of redemption from sin by LOVE. Celibacy is expedient for the aspirants in the East, as those lower races are soon to die out, but is contrary to the scheme of evolution for the West, because a new race is to be cradled here, and GENERATIVE PURITY is therefore the watchword of the Disciple in this part of the world. A new race is to be LOVED into existence, and thus the ills that now afflict humanity through generations of begettal in passion will cease; even Death will at last be overcome in the new dispensation, because the ethereal purity of the bodies will obviate necessity for renewal.

While there is much definite information about that age in the Bible, one point is shrouded in insoluble mystery: "The day knoweth no man, not even the Angels in Heaven, nor the Son." Christians in all ages since the Gospel was first preached have yearned for that day when the Sons of Light shall be manifest. The Father alone, being Highest Initiate among the Lords of Mind, is able to foresee the time when the separative, self-seeking mind will yield to the self-negating, unifying spirit of love. One point is very clear, however: It will be just as impossible for anyone to live under the conditions of the New Heaven and the New Earth who has not the properly constituted body, called "Wedding Garment" in the Bible, as it was for the degenerate Atlanteans who lacked lungs to breathe when the atmospheric change came.

It is a scientific fact that the state of the blood affects the mind and vice versa. A sound body is therefore indispensable to sane mentality. Only a sane mind can transcend passion; only a sound body can generate another that is as pure. The ROSICRUCIANS have aimed to heal the body that it may harbor a sane mind and a pure love, for each conception under those conditions is a step toward the day of the lord for which we all long so ardently. This is the reason for the healing activities, and it is the meaning of our motto, "A Sane Mind, a Soft Heart, a Sound Body."

It has been written in various works that the members of the order took a vow to heal others free of charge. This statement is somewhat garbled. The lay brothers took a vow to MINISTER to all according to the best of their ability FREE OF CHARGE. That vow included healing, of course, in the case of such men as Paracelsus, who had ability in that direction; by the combination method of physical remedies applied under favorable stars and spiritual counsel he was highly successful. Others were not suited to be healers but labored in other directions, BUT ALL WERE ALIKE IN ONE PARTICULAR--THEY NEVER CHARGED FOR THEIR SERVICES, and they labored in secret without flourish of trumpet or sound of drum.

Christ gave two commands to His messengers: "Preach the Gospel" (of the coming Age) and "Heal the sick." One is as binding as the other, and, for the foregoing reasons, as necessary. To comply with the second command the Elder Brothers have evolved a system of healing which combines the best points in the various schools of today with a method of diagnosis and treatments as certain as it is simple, and thus a long step has been taken to lift the art of healing from the sands of experiment to the rock of exact knowledge.

It is a true, good and valid reason when we say that we want to help others for Christ's sake. He is now immured in the Earth, groaning and travailing and waiting for liberation. Pain and sickness are caused by transgression of the laws of life, therefore, they crystallize the dense body, give a firmer grip on the vital body and retard the day of our liberation, as well as His. By helping the sick to attain health and by teaching them to live in harmony with the laws of life so that they may maintain health, we are hastening the day of His coming. May God bless our efforts and strengthen our hands in the Good Work.

THE INVISIBLE HELPERS:

Our method of healing is not altogether a spiritual matter. We use physical means wherever it is possible. There are times even when we send our patients to a doctor in order that they may obtain quick relief from him by a certain treatment which we cannot give as promptly by other methods. Also, the diet of patients receives careful attention, for naturally, as the body is built up of physical substances, we are giving medicine by using the right food. But in addition, healing is carried on by the Elder Brothers through a band of Invisible Helpers whom they are instructing.

These Invisible Helpers are Probationers who during the daytime live a worthy life of helpfulness and thereby fit themselves or earn for themselves the privilege of being helpful through the instrumentality of the Elder Brothers at night. These Probationers are gathered together in bands according to their temperaments and ability. They are under instruction of other Probationers who are doctors, and all of them work under the guidance of the Elder Brothers, who naturally are the moving Spirits in the whole work.

The system of forming and organizing a band of Invisible Helpers is accomplished by the use of the effluvia from their vital bodies. The first of this is obtained at the time when the probationer signs his obligation and it is renewed every day when he makes the record upon his report blank. So long as he is faithful and lives the life of purity and service it forms an unbroken link between him and the ELDER BROTHERS. Each group of healers usually consists of twelve

Probationers besides their instructor and they are generally taken from the same locality because the night is the same for them all. It would not be feasible to group one living in Australia with one living in Alaska for one would be going about his daily work while the other is taking his nightly rest. But people taken from almost anywhere in North or South America spend about the identical hours in rest and recuperation and these Probationers are then grouped according to their rising signs so that they may form a complete circle.

Regarding the system used to find those who have written to Headquarters for help, the same method is followed as in finding the Probationers. That is to say, applicants for relief are required to write the letter of request with pen and ink. Thus the paper is impregnated with a part of their vital body and this is taken from the letter by the Elder Brothers. It contains an accurate gauge of the condition of the individual from whom it came and it also acts as an "open sesame" to the Helpers who are given charge of this case. Through that they have free access to his body, and a considerable number of patients who come for healing write that they have both seen and felt the Helpers working both inside and outside their bodies. As the condition of the patient changes so does the record. Therefore the patients are required to write with pen and ink a few words every week and mail it to Headquarters. Thus the Elder Brothers are in constant touch with their condition and are able to direct intelligently the work of restoration to health.

This work never ceases. It is continuous, as the Sun is always absent from a part of the globe and the Probationers in that part are active in the work of healing and helping during the hours of bodily rest.

Anatomically man belongs to the mammals, whose blood corpuscles are not nucleated. The nuclei found in the blood of lower animals are the vantage ground of the Group Spirits, but the higher animals are so far advanced upon the road to individualization that their blood is free from this influence. In the fetus where the mother acts as a Group Spirit for the first few weeks, she nucleates the blood, but as soon as the Ego begins work, the first thing it does is to disintegrate these nucleated blood corpuscles, and at the time of the quickening not a single such corpuscle remains. The Ego is master of its vehicle, a heritage which no one may take from it under any pretense whatever. To do so is black magic, whether the person knows it or not, and though the benevolent motive would of course have a certain mitigating effect in another direction, the fat nevertheless remains that one is upon dangerous ground when attempting to meddle with the blood of anyone who does not desire it and who has not asked for such treatment.

There is only one exception to this rule. Children until the age of puberty are, so to say, a part of their parents, because there is stored in the thymus gland an essence of the parental blood which the child uses in manufacturing its own supply during the years of childhood, while the desire body is in the course of gestation. As time goes on the supply in the thymus gland becomes smaller and smaller and the child attains more and more to a realization of its own individuality. By the time the thymus gland has disappeared the desire body has matured sufficiently to take part in the alchemy of transmuting the Saturnine skeleton into the Jupiterian vehicle which will thus incorporate the essence of the present physical body. Interference with the blood stops this process; therefore it is only until the time of puberty that the parent may at for the child in giving the ether which admits the Invisible Helper.

The greatest drawback to our healing activity comes from the negligence of patients. Our requirements are very simple. We only ask them to write once a week with pen and ink, so that the etheric effluvia coming from the hand during writing may furnish our Invisible Helpers with a key of admission to the patient's system. But simple as is this rule, some fail to write. Here is a case where a person who had for many years had vertebrae displaced and who was cured by our treatment, though osteopaths, chiropractors, and several others who had tried, had found it impossible to replace these vertebrae. The poor man was therefore in constant pain and sick in bed most of the time, entirely unable to work. The treatment of our Invisible Helpers replaced the vertebrae, and they are still in place. The man went to work and it seemed wonderful. But becoming so elated at the idea that he was so entirely free, he disregarded our instruction to keep on writing, so that our Invisible helpers might have the chance to keep his vertebrae in place for a sufficient length of time till they would stay put. Now comes the following letter showing that we were right in requesting him to do this, and he did wrong not to obey. He says: "A short time ago I wrote that I was cured, and would discontinue my weekly letters, but I see now that I have made a big mistake. Since then my back has pained me nearly all the time and I am getting round-shouldered again, though the vertebrae are in place where the injury was. It seems as though I am asking a lot of you to take this up the second time, but I did not realize the influence the Invisible Helpers had over me and how much I was dependent on them."

THE SPIRITUAL PANACEA:

In the coming of the Christ to Earth we have an analogy between it and the administering of the spiritual Panacea, according to the law, "As above, so below." There is in every little cell of the human body a separate cell life, but over and above that is the Ego which directs and controls all cells so that they act in harmony. During certain protracted illnesses the Ego becomes so intent upon the suffering that it ceases to vivify the cells fully; thus bodily ailment breeds mental inaction and it may become impossible to throw off disease without a special impulse to dispel the mental fog and start the cell activities anew. That is what the spiritual Panacea does. As the inrushing Christ Life on Golgotha commenced to dispel the shell of fear bred by inexorable law that hung like a pall about the Earth; as it started the millions of human beings upon the path of peace and good will, so also when the Panacea is applied does the concentrated Christ Life therein contained rush through the patient's body and infuse each cell with a rhythm that awakens the imprisoned Ego from its lethargy and gives back life and health.

In order to describe the Panacea an experience of the author will be related: A substance was shown to him in the Temple of the Rosicrucians on a certain memorable night, with which the Universal Spirit could be combined as readily as great quantities of ammonia combine with water. Three spheres were suspended one above the other in the center of the Temple, the middle sphere being about half way between the floor and ceiling. It was much larger than the other two, which hung one above and one below. Inside the large central sphere was a smaller contained which held a number of packages filled with that substance. When the Brothers had placed themselves in certain positions, when the harmony of certain music had prepared the way, suddenly the three globes began to glow with the three primary colors, blue, yellow, and red. To the vision of the writer it was plain how during the incantation of the formula the container having in it the before mentioned packages became aglow with a spiritual essence that was not there before. Some of these were later used by the Brother with instantaneous success. Before them the crystallizing particles enveloping the spiritual centers of the patient scattered like magic, and the sufferer awoke to a recognition of physical health and well-being.

CHAPTER X

THE SCIENCE OF NUTRITION

GENERAL PRINCIPLES:

If we begin with the dense vehicle and consider the physical means available to improve it and make it the best possible instrument for the Spirit and afterward consider the spiritual means to the same end, we shall be including all the other vehicles as well; therefore we shall follow that method.

The first visible state of a human embryo is a small, globulous, pulpy or jelly-like substance, similar to albumen, or the white of an egg. In this pulpy globule various particles of more solid matter appear. These gradually increase in bulk and density until they come in contact with one another. The different points of contact are slowly modified into joints or hinges and thus a distinct framework of solid matter, a skeleton, is gradually formed.

During the formation of this framework the surrounding pulpy matter accumulates and changes in form until at length that degree of organization develops which is known as a fetus. This becomes larger, firmer, and more fully organized up to the time of birth, when the stage of infancy begins.

The same process of consolidation which commenced with the first visible stage of existence, still continues. The being passes through the different stages of infancy, childhood, youth, manhood or womanhood, old age, and at last comes to the change that is called death.

Each of these stages is characterized by an INCREASING DEGREE OF HARDNESS AND SOLIDITY.

There is a gradual increase in density and firmness of the bones, tendons, cartilages, ligaments, tissues, membranes, the coverings and even the very substance of the stomach, liver, lungs, and other organs. The joints become rigid and dry. They begin to crack and grate when they are moved, because the synovial fluid, which oils and softens them, is diminished in quantity and rendered too thick and glutinous to serve that purpose.

The heart, the brain, and the entire muscular system, spinal cord, nerves, eyes, etc., partake of the same consolidating process, growing more and more rigid. Millions upon millions of the minute capillary vessels which ramify and spread like the branches of a tree throughout the entire body, gradually choke up and change into solid fiber, no longer pervious to the blood.

The larger blood vessels, both arteries and veins, indurate, lose their elasticity, grow smaller, and become incapable of carrying the required amount of blood. The fluids of the body thicken and become putrid, loaded with earthy matter. The skin withers and grows wrinkled and dry. The hair falls out for lack of oil. The teeth decay and drop out for lack of gelatin. The motor nerves begin to dry up and the movements of the body become awkward, and slow. The senses fail; the circulation of the blood is retarded; it stagnates and congeals in the vessels. More and more the body loses its former powers. Once elastic, healthy, alert, pliable, active, and sensitive, it becomes rigid, slow, and insensible. Finally, it dies of old age.

The question now arises, What is the cause of this gradual ossification of the body, bringing rigidity, decrepitude and death?

From the purely physical standpoint, chemists seem to be unanimous in the opinion that it is principally an increase of phosphate of lime (bone matter), carbonate of lime (common chalk), and sulphate of lime (plaster of Paris), with occasionally a little magnesia and an insignificant amount of other earthy matters.

The only difference between the body of old age and that of childhood is the greater density, toughness and rigidity, caused by the greater proportion of calcareous, earthy matter entering into the composition of the former. The bones of a child are composed of three parts of gelatin to one part of earthy matter. In old age this proportion is reversed. What is the source of this death-dealing accumulation of solid matter?

It seems to be axiomatic that the entire body is nourished by the blood and that everything contained in the body, of whatever nature, has first been in the blood. Analysis shows that the blood holds earthy substances of the same kind as the solidifying agents--and mark!--the ARTERIAL blood contains more earthy matter than the VENOUS blood.

This is highly important. It shows that in every cycle the blood deposits earthy substances. It is therefore the common carrier that chokes up the system. But its supply of earthy matter must be replenished; otherwise it could not continue to do this. Where does it renew its deadly load? There can be but one answer to that question--from the food and drink; there is absolutely no other source.

The food and drink which nourish the body must be, at the same time, the primary source of the calcareous, earthy matter which is deposited by the blood all over the system, causing decrepitude and finally death. To sustain physical life it is necessary that we eat and drink, but as there are many kinds of food and drink, it behooves us, in the light of the above facts, to ascertain, if possible, what kinds contain the smallest proportion of destructive matter. If we can find such food we can lengthen our lives, and from an occult standpoint, it is desirable to live as long as possible in each dense body, particularly after a start has been made toward the path. So many years are required to educate, through childhood and hot youth, each body inhabited, until the Spirit can at least obtain some control over it, that the longer we retain a body that has become amenable to the Spirit's promptings, the better. Therefore it is highly important that the pupil partake of such food and drink only as will deposit the least amount of hardening matter and at the same time keep the excretory organs active.

The skin and the urinary system are the saviors of man from an early grave. Were it not that by their means, most of the earthy matter taken from our food is eliminated, no one would live ten years.

It has been estimated that ordinary, undistilled spring water contains carbonate and other compounds of lime to such an extent that the average quantity used each day by one person in the form of tea, coffee, soup, etc., would in forty years form a block of solid chalk or marble the size of a man. It is also a significant fact that although phosphate of lime is always found in the urine of adults, it is not found in the urine of children, because in them the rapid formation of bone requires that this salt be retained. During the period of gestation there is very little earthy matter in the urine of the mother, as it is used in the building of the fetus. In ordinary circumstances, however, earthy matter is very much in evidence in the urine of adults and to this we owe the feat that physical life reaches even its present length.

Undistilled water, when taken internally, is man's worst enemy, but used externally, it becomes his best friend. It keeps the pores of the skin open, induces circulation of the blood and prevents the stagnation which affords the best opportunity for the depositing of the earthy, death-dealing phosphate of lime.

Harvey, who discovered the circulation of the blood, said that health denotes a free circulation and disease is the result of an obstructed circulation of the blood.

The bathtub is a great aid in keeping up the health of the body and should be freely used the aspirant to the higher life. Perspiration, sensible and insensible, carries more earthy matter out of the body than any other agency.

As long as fuel is supplied and the fire kept free from ashes, it will burn. The kidneys are important in carrying away the ashes from the body, but despite the great amount of earthy matter carried away by urine, enough remains in many cases to form gravel and stone in the bladder, causing untold agony and often death.

Let no one be deceived into thinking that water contains less stone because it has been boiled. The stone that forms on the bottom of the teakettle has been left there by the evaporated water which escaped from the kettle as steam. If the steam were condensed, we should have distilled water, which is an important adjunct in keeping the body young.

There is absolutely no earthy matter in distilled water, nor in rain water, snow or hail (except what may be gathered in contact with house-tops, etc.), but coffee, tea, or soup made with ordinary water, no matter how long boiled, is not purified of the earthy particles; on the contrary, the longer they are boiled, the more heavily charged with ash they become. Those suffering from urinary diseases should never drink any but distilled water.

It may be said generally of the solid foods we take into our systems, that fresh vegetables and ripe fruits contain the greatest proportion of nutritious matter and the least of earthy substances.

Proper food given at the right time and under the right conditions will not only cure but prevent disease.

It is popularly supposed that sugar or any saccharine substance is injurious to the general health, and particularly to the teeth, causing their decay and the resulting toothache. Only under certain circumstances is this true. It is harmful in certain diseases, such as biliousness and dyspepsia, or if held long in the mouth as candy, but if sparingly used during good health and the amount gradually increased as the stomach becomes accustomed to its use, it will be found very nourishing. The health of Negroes becomes greatly improved during the sugar-cane harvest time, notwithstanding their increased labor. This is attributed solely to their fondness for the sweet cane-juice. The same may be said of horses, cows, and other animals in those localities, which are all fond of the refuse syrup fed to them. They grow fat in harvest time, their coats becoming sleek and shining. Horses fed on boiled carrots for a few weeks will get a coat like silk, owing to the saccharine juices of that vegetable. Sugar is a nutritious and beneficial article of diet and contains no ash whatever.

Fruits are an ideal diet. They are in fact evolved by the tree to induce animal and man to eat them, so that the seed may be disseminated, as flowers entice bees for a similar purpose.

Fresh fruit contains water of the purest and best kind, capable of permeating the system in a marvelous manner. Grape juice is a particularly wonderful solvent. It thins and stimulates the blood, opening the way into capillaries already dried and choked up--if the process has not gone too far. By a course of unfermented grape juice treatment, people with sunken eyes, wrinkled skins and poor complexions become plump, ruddy, and lively. The increased permeability enables the Spirit to manifest more freely and with renewed energy.

Considering the body from a purely physical standpoint, it is what we might call a chemical furnace, the food being the fuel. The more the body is exercised, the ore fuel it requires. It would be foolish for a man to change an ordinary diet which for years had adequately nourished him, and take up a new method without due thought as to which would be the best for serving his purpose. To simply eliminate meats from the ordinary diet of meat-eaters would unquestionably undermine the health of most persons. The only safe way is to experiment and study the matter out first, using due discrimination. No fixed rules can be given, the matter of diet being as individual as any other characteristic. All that can be done is to describe the general influence of each chemical element, allowing the aspirant to work out his own method.

Neither must we allow the appearance of a person to influence our judgment as to the condition of his health. Certain general ideas of how a healthy person should look are commonly accepted, but there is no valid reason for so judging. Ruddy cheeks might be an indication of health in one individual and of disease in another. There is no particular rule by which good health can be known except the feeling of comfort and well-being which is enjoyed by the individual himself, irrespective of appearances.

Water is the great solvent.

Nitrogen or protein is the essential builder of flesh, but contains some earthy matter.

Carbohydrates or sugars are the principle power-producers.

Fats are the producers of heat and the storers of reserve force.

Ash is mineral, earthy, and chokes the system. We need have no fear of not obtaining it in sufficient quantities to build the bones; on the contrary, we cannot be too careful to get as little as possible.

The calorie is the simple unit of heat. In a pound of Brazil nuts, for instance, when bought at the market, 49.6 per cent of the whole is waste (shells), but the remaining 50.4 per cent contains 1485 calories. That means that about one-half of what is bought is waste, but the remainder contains the number of calories named. That we may get the nearest amount of strength from our food we must pay attention to the number of calories it contains, for from them we obtain the energy required to perform our daily work.

Chocolate is the most nutritious food we have; also cocoa, in its powdered state, is the most dangerous of all foods, containing three times as much ash as most of the others, and ten times as much as many. It is a powerful food and also a powerful poison, for it chokes the system more quickly than any other substance.

Of course, it will require some study at first to secure the best nourishment, but it pays in health and longevity and secures the free use of the body, making study and application to higher things possible. After a while one will become so familiar with the subject that he will need to give it no particular attention.

It must be remembered that not all of the chemical substances contained in each article of food are available for use in the system, because there are certain portions which the body refuses to assimilate.

Of vegetables we digest only about 83 per cent of the proteins, 90 per cent of the fat, and 95 per cent of the carbohydrates.

Of fruits we assimilate about 85 per cent of the proteins, 90 per cent of the fat, and 90 per cent of the carbohydrates.

Phosphorous is the particular element by means of which the Ego is able to express thought and influence the dense physical body. It is also a fact that the proportion and variation of this substance is found to correspond to the state and stage of intelligence of the individual. Idiots have very little phosphorus; shrewd thinkers have much; and in the animal world, the degree of consciousness and intelligence is in proportion to the amount of phosphorus contained in the brain.

It is therefore of great importance that the aspirant who is to use his body for mental and spiritual work, should supply his brain with the substance necessary for that purpose. Most vegetables and fruits contain a certain amount of phosphorus, but it is a peculiar fat that the greater proportion is contained in the leaves, which are usually thrown away. It is found in considerable quantities in grapes, onions, sage, beans, cloves, pineapples, in the leaves and stalks of many vegetables, and also in sugar-cane juice, but not in refined sugar.

The following table shows the proportions of phosphoric acid in a few articles:

100,000 parts of:

Barley, dry, contains of phosphoric acid.........210   parts

Beans 292   "

Beets 167   "

Beets, Leaves of................................690   "

Buckwheat.......................................170   "

Carrots, dry..395   "

Carrots, Leaves of..............................963   "

Linseed...880   "

Linseed, Stalks of..............................118   "

Parsnips..111   "

Parsnips, Leaves of............................1784   "

Peas 190   "

In conclusion, let the aspirant choose such food as is most easily digested, for the more easily the energy in food is extracted, the longer time will the system have for recuperation before it becomes necessary to replenish the supply. Milk should never be drunk as one may drink a glass of water. Taken in that way, it forms in the stomach a large cheese ball, quite impervious to the action of the gastric juices. It should be sipped for it will then form many small globules in the stomach, which are easily assimilated. Citrus fruits are powerful antiseptics, and cereals, particularly rice, are antitoxins of great efficiency.

Having now explained, from the purely material point of view, what is necessary for the dense body, we will consider the subject from the occult side, taking into consideration the effect on the two invisible bodies which interpenetrate the dense body.

The particular stronghold of the desire body is in the muscles and the cerebrospinal nervous system, as already shown. The energy displayed by a person when laboring under great excitement or anger is an example of this. At such times the whole muscular system is tense and no hard labor is so exhausting as a "fit of temper." It sometimes leaves the body prostrated for weeks. There can be seen the necessity for improving the desire body by controlling the temper, thus sparing the dense body the suffering resulting from the ungoverned action of the desire body.

Looking at the matter from an occult standpoint, all consciousness in the Physical World is the result of the constant war between the desire and vital bodies.

The tendency of the vital body is to soften and build. Its chief expression is the blood and the glands, also the sympathetic nervous system, having obtained ingress into the stronghold of the desire body (the muscular and the voluntary nervous systems) when it began to develop the heart into a voluntary muscle.

The tendency of the desire body is to harden, and it in turn has invaded the realm of the vital body, gaining possession of the spleen and making the white blood corpuscles, which are not "the policemen of the system" as science now thinks, but destroyers. It uses the blood to carry these tiny destroyers all over the body. They pass through the walls of arteries and veins whenever annoyance is felt, and especially in times of great anger. Then the rush of forces in the desire body makes the arteries and veins swell and opens the way for the passage of the white corpuscles into the tissues of the body, where they form bases for the earthy matter which kills the body.

Given the same amount and kind of food, the person of serene and jovial disposition will live longer, enjoy better health, and be more active than the person who worries, or loses his temper. The latter will make and distribute through his body more destructive white corpuscles than the former. Were a scientist to analyze the bodies of these two men, he would find that there was considerably less earthy matter in the body of the kindly disposed man than in that of the scold.

This destruction is constantly going on and it is not possible to keep all the destroyers out, nor is such the intention. If the vital body had uninterrupted sway, it would build and build, using all the energy for that purpose. There would be no consciousness and thought. It is because the desire body checks and hardens the inner parts that consciousness develops.

There was a time in the far, far past when we set out the concretions, as do the mollusks, leaving the body soft, flexible, and boneless, but at that time we had only the dull, glimmering consciousness the mollusks now have. Before we could advance, it became necessary to retain the concretions and it will be found that the stage of consciousness of any species in in proportion to the development of the bony framework WITHIN. The Ego must have the solid bones with the semi-fluid red marrow, in order to be able to build the red blood corpuscles for its expression. That is the highest development of the dense body.

REASONS FOR A VEGETARIAN DIET:

Most people feel that a meal without meat is incomplete, for from time immemorial it has been regarded as an axiom that meat is the most strengthening food we have. All other foodstuffs have been looked upon as mere accessories to the one or more kinds of flesh on the menu. Nothing could be more erroneous; science has proved by experiments that invariable the nourishment obtained from vegetables has a greater sustaining power, and the reason is easy to see when we look into the matter from the occult side.

The law of assimilation is that "no particle of food may be built into the body by the forces whose task that is until it has been overcome by the in-dwelling spirit," because he must be absolute and undisputed ruler in the body, governing the cell lives as an autocrat, or they would each go their own way as they do in decay when the Ego has fled.

It is evident that the dimmer the consciousness of a cell is, the easier it is to overpower it, and the longer it will remain in subjection. The different kingdoms have different vehicles and consequently a different consciousness. The mineral has only its dense body and a consciousness like the deepest trance. It would therefore be easiest to subject foods taken directly from the mineral kingdom. Mineral food would remain with us the longest, obviating the necessity of Eating so often; but unfortunately we find that the human organism vibrates so rapidly that it is incapable of assimilating the inert mineral directly. Salt and like substances are passed out of the system at once without having been assimilated at all; the air is full of nitrogen which we need to repair waste, we breathe it into our system, yet cannot assimilate it or any other mineral till it has first been transmuted in Nature's laboratory and built into the plants.

The plants have a dense and a vital body, which enables them to do this work; their consciousness is as a deep, dreamless sleep. Thus it is easy for the Ego to overpower the vegetable cells and keep them in subjection for a long time, hence the great sustaining power of the vegetable.

In animal food the cells have already become more individualized, and as the animal has a desire body giving it a passional nature, it is easily understood that when we eat meat it is harder to overcome these cells which have animal consciousness resembling the dream state, and also that such particles will not stay long in subjection, hence a meat diet requires larger quantities and more frequent meals than the vegetable or fruit diet. If we should go one step farther and eat the flesh of carnivorous animals, we should find ourselves hungry all the time, for there the cells have become exceedingly individualized and will therefore seek their freedom and gain it so much the quicker. That this is so, is well illustrated in the case of the wolf, the vulture, and the cannibal, which have become proverbs for hunger, and as the human liver is too small to take care of even the ordinary meat diet, it is evident that if the cannibal lived solely upon human flesh instead of using it as an occasional "tidbit," he would soon succumb, for while too much of the carbohydrates, sugars, starches, and fats do little if any harm to the system, being exhaled through the lungs as carbonic acid gas or passing as water by way of the kidneys and the skin, an excess of meat is also burned up, but leaves poisonous uric acid and it is being more and more recognized that the less meat we eat the better for our well-being.

It is natural that we should desire the very best of food, but every animal body has in it the poisons of decay. The venous blood is filled with carbon dioxide and other noxious products on their way to the kidneys or the pores of the skin to be expelled as urine or perspiration. These loathsome substances are in every part of the flesh and when we eat such food we are filling our own bodies with toxic poisons. Much sickness is due to our use of flesh foods.

There is plenty of proof that a carnivorous diet fosters ferocity. We may mention the well-known fierceness of beasts of prey and the cruelty of the meat-eating American Indian as fair examples. On the other hand, the prodigious strength and the docile nature of the ox, the elephant, and the horse show the effects of the herb diet on animals, while the vegetarian and peaceable nations of the Orient are a proof of the correctness of the argument against a flesh diet which cannot successfully be gainsaid.

As soon as we adopt the vegetarian diet, we escape one of the most serious menaces of health, namely the putrefaction of particles of flesh imbedded between the teeth, and this is not one of the least arguments why a vegetarian diet should be adopted. Fruits, cereals, and vegetables are from their very natures SLOW TO DECAY, each particle contains an enormous amount of ether which keeps it alive and sweet for a long time, whereas the ether which interpenetrated the flesh and composed the vital body of an animal, was taken away with the Spirit thereof at the time of death. Thus the danger from infection through vegetable food is very small in the first place, but many of them so far from being poisonous, are actually antiseptic in a very high degree. This applies particularly to the citrus fruits: oranges, lemons, grapefruit, etc., not to speak of the king of all antiseptics, the pineapple, which has been used very often with complete success as a cure for the dreaded diphtheria, which is only another name for a septic sore throat. Thus instead of poisoning the digestive tract with putrefactive elements as meats do, FRUITS CLEANSE AND PURIFY THE SYSTEM, and the pineapple is one of the superior to pepsin, and no fiendish cruelty is used to obtain it.

There are twelve salts in the body; they are very vital and represent the twelve signs of the zodiac. These salts are required for the building of the body. They are not mineral salts as generally supposed, but are vegetable. The mineral has no vital body, and it is only by way of the vital body that assimilation is accomplished; therefore, we have to obtain these salts through the vegetable kingdom.

Doctors claim to do this, but they are not aware that fire used in the process drives out and destroys the vital body of the plant just as cremation treats our body, and leaves only the mineral parts. Therefore, if we desire to renew the supply of any salt in our body we must obtain it from the UNCOOKED plant. To the sick this is the way it should be administered.

But we must not jump to the conclusion that everyone should quit eating meat and live on raw plant life. At our present stage of evolution there are very few who can do so. We must take care not to raise the vibrations of our bodies too rapidly, for we, to continue our labor among present conditions, must have a body fitted for the work, but let us keep the thought always with us.

There is in the skull at the base of the brain a flame. It burns continually in the medulla oblongata at the head of the spinal cord, and like the fire on the altar of the tabernacle, is of divine origin. This fire emits a singing sound like the buzz of a bee, which is the keynote of the physical body, and is sounded by the archetype. It builds in and cements together that mass of cells known as "our body."

The fire burns high or low, clear or dim, according to how we feed it. There is fire in everything in nature EXCEPT THE MINERAL KINGDOM. It has no vital body and therefore no avenue for the ingress of the Life Spirit, the fire. We replenish this sacred fire partly from the FORCES FROM THE SUN entering the vital body through the etheric counterpart of the spleen and from there to the solar plexus where it is colored and then carried upward through the blood. We also FEED THE FIRE FROM THE LIVING FIRE WE ABSORB FROM THE UNCOOKED FOOD WHICH WE EAT AND THUS ASSIMILATE.

Looking at the matter of flesh-eating from the ethical side also, it is against the higher conception to kill to eat. In olden times man went out to the chase as any beast of prey, rough and callous; now he does his hunting in the butcher shop, where none of the nauseating sights of the slaughter house will sicken him. If each had to go into those blood places where horrors are enacted day after day to be able to satisfy an abnormal injurious habit which causes more sickness and suffering than even liquor craving; if each had to wield the bloody knife and plunge it into the quivering flesh of his victim, how much meat would we eat? Very little. In order to escape doing this nauseating work ourselves on occasion, we force a fellow being to stand in that bloody pen day after day killing thousands of animals every day of the wee; we brutalize him to such an extent that the law will not allow him to sit on a jury in a capital case because he has ceased to have any regard for life.

The animals which we kill also cry aloud against this murder; there is a cloud of gloom and hatred over the great slaughter cities. The law protects cats and dogs against cruelty. We all rejoice to see the little squirrels in the city parks come and take food from our hands, but as soon as there is money in the flesh or fur of an animal, man ceases to have regard for its right to live, and becomes its most dangerous foe, feeding and breeding it for gain, imposing suffering and hardships upon a fellow being for the sake of gold. We have a heavy debt to pay to the lower creatures whose mentors we should be; whose murderers we are, and the good law which works every to correct abuses will also in time relegate the habit of Eating murdered animals to the scrapheap of obsolete practices as cannibalism is now.

It is the nature of a beast of prey to eat any animal that comes in its path, and its organs are such that it must have that kind of a diet to exist, but EVERYTHING IS IN A STAGE OF BECOMING; it is always changing to something higher. Man, in his earlier stages of unfoldment, was also like the beasts of prey in certain respects; however, he is to become God-like and thus he must cease to destroy at some time in order that he may commence to create. Flesh food has fostered human ingenuity of a low order in the past; it has served a purpose in our evolution; but we are now standing on the threshold of a new age when self-sacrifice and service will bring spiritual growth to humanity. The evolution of the mind will bring a wisdom beyond our greatest conception, but before it will be safe to entrust us with that wisdom, we must become HARMLESS as doves, for otherwise we should be apt to turn it to such selfish and destructive purposes that it would be an inconceivable menace to our fellow men. To avoid this the vegetarian diet must be adopted.

We have been taught that there is no life in the universe but the life of God; that "in Him we live and move and have our being"; that His life animates everything that is, and therefore we naturally understand that as soon as we take LIFE we are destroying FORM built by God for his manifestation. The lower animals are evolving Spirits and have sensibilities. It is their desire for experience that causes them to build their various FORMS, and when we take their forms away from them we deprive them of their opportunity for gaining experience. We hinder their evolution instead of helping them, and the day will come when we shall feel a deep disgust at the thought of making our stomachs the burying ground for the carcasses of murdered animals. All true Christians will be abstainers from flesh foods out of pure compassion; they will realize that all life is God's life, and to cause suffering to any sentient being is wrong.

In a great many places where the Bible speaks of "meat," it is very plain that flesh food is not meant. The chapter in Genesis where man's food is first allotted to him says that he should eat of every tree and herb bearing seed, "and to you it shall be for meat." The most evolved people at all times have abstained from flesh foods. We see, for instance, Daniel, who was a holy man and a wise man, beg that he might not be forced to eat meat, but that he and his companions be given pulse. The children of Israel in the wilderness are spoken of as "lusting after flesh," and their God is angry with them in consequence.

There is an esoteric meaning to the feeding of the multitude where fish was used as food, but looking to the purely material aspect we may sum up the points in our answer by reiterating that we shall some time outgrow flesh and fish Eating as we have risen above cannibalism. Whatever license may have been given in the barbaric past will disappear in the altruistic future, when more refined sensibilities shall have awakened us to a fuller sense of the horrors involved in the gratification of a carnivorous taste.

NECESSITY FOR AN ATTRACTIVE, BALANCED DIET:

In the most sublime of all prayers, we are taught by the Christ to pray for our daily bread, but under existing modern conditions, alas, how often do we get a stone instead.

Because of our complex civilization, of cold storage methods, and other abominations our food is such that, generally speaking, instead of nourishing the body as it should, it depletes us and makes us subject to various diseases; "indigestible" is a very mild arraignment of the food supply in most places where the public eats.

Even in the home, that which is placed upon the table to nourish and sustain and build the body in health, is often only an apology for food, masquerading under various seasonings and dressings as palatable, for we eat usually to please our palate rather than to nourish our bodies.

On the other hand, there is no denying that some people who profess to cook along scientific lines and with common sense, who profess to be vegetarians and are very strict in their notions of how food should be prepared, seem to lack all appreciation of the fact that food may be made palatable as well as wholesome and nutritious, that there is no incompatibility between the requirements of proper cooking and the pleasure afforded to the palate. Indeed it may be said that unless food is so cooked that it is pleasing to the palate as well as wholesome and nutritious, it falls far short of its full purpose. The palate has been given to us so that we may enjoy our food, that we may, as it were, receive it with gladness and welcome it into our body, for this furthers assimilation and nutrition, whereas unpalatable food is obnoxious to the recipient and therefore not so easily assimilated. This fact should be kept before the mind: It is not how much we eat that counts, but how much we assimilate.

Some who have been improperly instructed in this most important subject of nutrition may have been told that the legumes, peas, beans, etc., will take the place of meat, and they then commenced to devour these vegetables in great quantities after discarding meat. It is perfectly true that beans contain more protein than beefsteak, but the protein contained in the bean is not so readily assimilated. There is heavy waste and also uric acid in such foods that should be reckoned with, for unless counteracted by plenty of green vegetables, disastrous results are bound to follow. It is important to remember, however, that the green vegetables should not be eaten at the same meal with the heavy legumes. There are others who, after leaving the meat diet, start to live on bread, potatoes, and similar starchy foods, with the result that they become undernourished and anemic. A satisfactory diet must be properly balanced in every respect, and only in so far as we study the system of diet required to keep our body in good health can we expect to obtain the proper results.

Diet, like health, is determined individually, and no general standard can be set up. At the same time, it may be safely said that the less meat we can get along with, the better our general health will be. But if we wish to without it altogether, it is absolutely essential that we should study a table of food values so that we get the necessary proteins from the vegetables we eat. No man can go to the ordinary table and get sufficient nourishment if he eats only the vegetables provided as accessories to the meat; he must have beans, peas, nuts, and like foods which are rich in protein to take the place of the discarded flesh, or he will starve.

THE ROLE OF STIMULANTS IN EVOLUTION:

The spirit alcohol, which is fermented OUTSIDE the system, is being superseded by sugar, which ferments WITHIN. In the past a stimulant was indispensable in rousing the human Spirit from the lethargy attendant upon a meat diet; the bacchanalian orgies in ancient temples, which properly fill us with horror nowadays, were then of immense value in human development. As consumption of sugar increases, use of alcohol diminishes and, concurrently, the moral standard is gradually elevated. People grow more altruistic and Christ-like in proportion to their use of the non- inebriating stimulant, and therefore the temperance movement is one of the most powerful factors to hasten the coming of Christ.

It is evident that evolutionary progress is elevating the lower kingdoms as well as humanity. The animals, particularly the domesticated species, are nearing individualization, and their withdrawal from manifestation has already commenced. As a result it will in time be impossible to obtain flesh food. Then the death knell of "King Alcohol" will have struck, for only flesh eaters crave liquor.

In the meantime plant life is growing more sentient. The lateral limbs of trees produce more abundantly than do vertical branches because in plants, as in us, consciousness results from the antagonistic activities of the desire and vital currents. Lateral limbs are swept through their entire length by desire currents which circle our planet and which act so powerfully in the horizontal animal spines. The desire currents rouse the sleeping plant life in the lateral limbs to a higher degree of consciousness than is the case with the vertical branches, which are traversed lengthwise by vital currents radiating from the center of the Earth. Thus, in time, the plants will also become too sensitive as food and another source must be sought.

Today, we have considerable ability in working with the chemical mineral substances; we mold them into houses, ships, and all outer things which evidence our civilization. We are masters of the minerals OUTSIDE our body, but powerless to assimilate and use them INSIDE our system to build our organs until the plant life has transmuted crystals into crystalloids. Our work with the minerals in the exterior world is raising their vibration and paving the way for direct interior use. By spiritual alchemy we shall build the temple of the Spirit, conquer the dust whence we came, and qualify as true Master Masons prepared for work in higher spheres.

FASTING AS A MEANS OF HEALING AND A FACTOR IN SOUL GROWTH:

We may readily conceive that there are more people in the West who die from overeating than from getting too little food. Under certain conditions fasting for a day or two is undoubtedly beneficial, but just as there are gourmands and gluttons, so there are others who go to the opposite extreme and fast to excess. There lies a great danger. The best way is to eat in moderation and to eat the proper kinds of food; then it will not be necessary to fast at all.

If we study the chemistry of food we shall find that certain foods have properties of value to the system under conditions of disorder, and taken properly food is really medicine. All the citrus fruits, for instance, are splendid antiseptics. THUS THEY PREVENT DISEASE. All the cereals, particularly rice, are antitoxins; they will kill disease and the germs of putrefaction. Thus, by knowing these medicinal properties of the different foods, we may very readily secure a supply of that which we need to cure our ordinary ailments by food instead of by fasting.

Under the ancient dispensations it was required that sacrifices of bulls and goats should be made as atonement for sin, for man then treasured his material possessions even higher than today, and felt keenly their loss when forced to give them up for such a purpose. Upon the altar of sacrifice men were forced to offer their cherished possessions for every transgression, God appearing to them as a hard taskmaster whose displeasure it was dangerous to incur. But there has always been an esoteric teaching, which is being promulgated exoterically today, and this teaching does not accept the sacrifice of an animal, money, or other possessions, but demands that each one make a sacrifice of himself. This was taught to the aspirants in the ancient Mystery School when they were prepared for the mystic rite of Initiation.

To them were explained the mysteries of the vital body, how it is composed of four ethers, etc. The aspirant was thoroughly instructed in the functions of the two lower ethers as compared with the two higher. He knew that all the purely animal functions of the body depended upon the density of the lower ethers, and that the two upper ethers composed the should body which was the vehicle of service. He aspired, naturally, to cultivate this glorious garment by self-abnegation, and by curbing the propensities of the lower nature, as we do today.

These facts were kept secret from the masses, as said, or rather they should have been, but some neophytes who were overzealous to attain, no matter how, forgot that it is only by service and unselfishness that the Golden Wedding Garment composed of the two higher ethers is grown. They thought that the occult maxim:

"Gold in the crucible,

Wrought in the fire;

Light as the winds,

Higher and higher"

meant only that so long as the lower nature, the dross, was expelled, it did not matter how, and if they could find an easy method, they would have left only the gold composed of the two higher ethers, the should body, in which they could enter the invisible world without let or hindrance. They reasoned that as the chemical ether is the agent of assimilation, it could be eliminated from the vital body by starving the physical vehicle.

But the result obtained by these misguided people and their followers was far from being what was intended by the training in the Mystery School. The candidate was there taught first and foremost that THE BODY IS THE TEMPLE OF GOD, and that to defile, destroy, or mutilate it in any manner is a great sin. Indulgence of the appetite is a sin, a defiling practice which brings with it certain retribution, but it is no more to be reprehended than the practice of fasting for soul growth. RIGHT LIVING IS NEITHER FASTING NOR FEASTING, but giving the body those elements which are necessary to maintain it in the proper form of health, strength, and efficiency as an instrument of the Spirit. Therefore fasting for soul growth is a pseudo-method which has exactly the opposite effect to that which it was designed to accomplish by its shortsighted originators.

THE HEALTH VALUE OF INDIGESTIBLE FOODS:

It may seem absurd, at the first blush, to say that the more indigestible our foods are the better the health will be; nevertheless, when the statement is slightly qualified, it is true. Foods which are usually reared as indigestible because we feel distress after Eating them, really cause trouble because they have been too thoroughly digested, while other foods which are nearly totally indigestible, and therefore in a sense not foods at all, leave us with all the feelings of health and well-being.

Lack of proper appreciation of these essential facts is at the bottom of the difficulties which many people experience when they adopt what they are pleased to call a vegetarian diet. They have in most cases suffered from digestive troubles before ceasing to eat flesh, and have in many cases adopted a fleshless diet with the expectation that they would work a miracle in restoring their health. They are therefore often bitterly disappointed that they feel no better, nay, in a number of cases they may even feel worse, because they continue their dietetic errors in all other respects, so that in many cases their reformed diet is from a standpoint of health, a thousand times worse than the usual mixed diet of the average person, and goodness knows, that is bad enough. In fact, instead of wondering that the body breaks down under the strain of dietetic indiscretion, it is really wonderful that it can stand up as well as it does in spite of the abuse and ill treatment to which it is subjected.

It happens not infrequently that people who apply to us for healing admit unblushingly the most atrocious dietetic blunders, perfectly oblivious to the fact that they are doing wrong. They will eat four to five meals a day, composed of hot cakes, coffee, eggs, beefsteak, white bread, potatoes, pie, cheese, etc., etc., and then they honestly wonder why they do not feel well. This class of people will claim that they have no bad habits. They smoke a few cigars, drink a few glasses of beer, or perhaps they take a cocktail or two; they live on what they call a "natural diet," go to bed at ten or eleven, and pat themselves on the back with the feeling that they are models. As a rule when it is first brought to their attention that they are committing serious blunders they stare in utter amazement and incredulity; they seem to doubt their senses when told that they are killing themselves with food; actually and in truth digging their graves with their teeth.

Nevertheless, that is absolutely true and it is not so much because their food is indigestible, either, as because of the lack of indigestible materials to mix among the highly concentrated foods which form the chief elements of such a diet. But in that respect that class of people are no worse than people who live on a diet of such concentrated foods as prunes, nuts, raisins, etc.

They also eat highly concentrated food; they get both protein from the nuts and carbohydrates from the raisins, but lack the indispensable though indigestible cellulose to give the necessary amount of bulk and cause irritation in the digestive tract which is absolutely essential to induce peristalsis and secretion of the necessary digestive ferments.

There is no question that whole wheat is much more nutritious, palatable, and healthful than white flour which is composed only of the starchy portions of the grain, but its health value is not particularly great because it is more easily digested than white bread, for as a matter of fact it is not, nor is the great benefit derived from whole wheat bread due to the mineral salts necessary to body building which it contains and which are absent in white bread. For it should be remembered that just as a portion of the protein contained in meat and the phosphorus contained in fish remain undigested, so also with the protein and phosphorus which abound in the whole meal bread. We do not assimilate all the protein and mineral salts which are contained in the coarsest portions of the whole wheat. But while the white bread is almost entirely digested and leaves but little ash, provided of course that it is well made, the coarser particles of the whole wheat flour pass through the intestinal tract undigested; they massage them, so to speak, irritate them and induce a flow of blood which keeps the intestines sweet and healthy. They do not pack as closely as the little residue left from highly concentrated foods, and therefore they take with them in the air spaces noxious gases, leaving the digestive tract pure and clean.

Compare the action on the bowels of such foods as eggs, and meat and cheese, which are almost totally assimilated and leave no coarse bulk to cleanse the bowels after a meal has been digested, with such vegetables as legumes (used sparingly), turnips, carrots, celery, onions, etc., which contain every element found in flesh and in addition the, to health, indispensable bulk composed of coarse fibrous matter which alone can sweep the intestinal tract, clear off all deleterious products of waste and leave the system in a healthy condition.

The archetype determines the form and figure of a person and this will be his normal statue in health, but by our dietetic disorder we often change this, so that the energy of the body is used in the process of eliminating an enormous amount of food which we cannot assimilate and therefore we grow thinner. The reverse happens when the eliminative powers are poor; then surplus flesh, or adipose tissue, is put on because of an unnatural diet. When a scientifically prepared diet is adopted, the people who have been too thin because of a previous wrong diet, taken on flesh, and conversely those who have put on unnatural flesh cease to do so and therefore their weight is reduced.

RESULTS OF EATING TOO FREQUENTLY:

Another fruitful cause of digestive disorders is the habit of Eating every few hours. People who are in the habit of Eating five or six times a day frequently assert that they are hungry and must have food or they are sick. As a matter of fact, the raving is due to a diseased condition of the stomach, and the relief results from the weight of food which deadens the stomach.

We call it criminal to give to a person addicted to the morphine habit more just because he craves it, and it would give temporary relief from suffering, and we should apply the same logic and philosophy to people who are poisoned by an excess of food. This is not theory, either, but the result of investigation which cannot be matched by experiments on animals or human beings, where the suffering incident to tabulating the results of investigations causes an unnatural digestive condition. There are no such barriers to one whose spiritual sight is opened and who can see the peristaltic action of the stomach and intestines when the system has been burdened. Then there exudes from the food a black poisonous gas which is thrown outward through the periphery of the aura by the man's vital body so long as he is in good health. But when his vitality becomes enfeebled and the flow of the solar force through the spleen is not as strong as usual, this poisonous gas remains around the abdominal region as a broad black band which poisons all organic activities of the body while it is there. When a person eats three meals a day there is a slight chance for the dissolution of the poison band generated by one meal before the next is taken. But where meals are eaten at intervals of only a few hours there is absolutely no chance for the person to rid himself of this poison cloud, and as a consequence he grows worse and worse, shortening the span of his natural life in a manner that would be a shocking surprise to most of these people could they realize it.

For these reasons anyone who wishes to obtain and maintain health should make it a point to eat only two or three times a day and SPARINGLY, taking care to secure an abundance of bulk rather than nutriment, for it is an actual fact that many, many more people die of too much nourishment of too little.

CHAPTER XI

ASTROLOGY AS AN AID TO HEALING

ASTROLOGICAL BASIS FOR HEALING:

It is well known to the modern physician that the condition of the blood, and therefore the condition of the whole body, changes in sympathy with the state of mind of the patient, and the more the physician uses suggestion as an adjunct to medicine the more successful he is. Few perhaps would credit the further fact that both our mental and physical condition is influenced by planetary rays which change as the planets move. In these days since the principle of radio-activity has been established we know that everybody projects into space numberless little particles. Wireless telegraphy has taught us that etheric waves travel swiftly and surely through space and operate a key according to our will. We also know that the rays of the sun affect us differently in the morning when they strike us horizontally than at noon when they are perpendicular. If the light rays from the swift-moving sun produce physical and mental changes, may not the persistent rays of slower planets also have an effect? If they have, they are factors in health not to be overlooked by a thoroughly scientific healer, and we therefore maintain that results may be obtained more easily at certain times when the stellar rays are propitious for the healing of a particular disease or for treatment with remedies previously prepared under auspicious conditions.

If physicians would study the science of astrology, they would thus with a very slight effort be able to diagnose their patient's condition in a manner altogether impossible from the ordinary diagnostician's point of view. Some physicians are waking up to that fact and have discovered by their experiences that the heavenly bodies do have an influence upon the human frame. For instance, when the writer was in Portland, Oregon, a physician mentioned as his observation that whenever it was possible for him to perform an operation while the moon was increasing in light, that is to say, going from the new to the full, the operation was always successful and no complications would set in. On the other hand, he had found that when circumstances compelled him to perform an operation when the Moon was going from the full to the dark there was great danger of trouble, and that such operations were never as satisfactory as those performed while the light of the Moon was increasing.

The way to find out the peculiarities of the Spirit that dwells in the patient's body is to cast his horoscope to see when the times are propitious for the administration of drugs, giving the appropriate HERBS at the proper time. Paracelsus did that, and therefore he was always successful with his patients; he never made a mistake. There are some who use astrology for that purpose today; the writer, for instance, has thus used it in diagnosis in many cases. He has then always been able to see the crises in the patient's condition, the past, present, and future; and thus has been able to afford much relief to persons suffering from various illnesses. It is to such uses that astrology should be put, and not degraded into fortune-telling for the sake of gold, for, like all spiritual sciences, it ought to be used for the benefit of humanity, regardless of mercenary considerations.

There are seven spheres, the planets of our solar system. Each has its own keynote and emits a sound varying from that of every other planet. One or more among them vibrates in particular synchrony with the seed atom of the Ego then seeking embodiment. This planet then corresponds to the "tonic" in the music scale, and though the tones from all the planets are necessary to build up an organism completely, each is modified and made to conform to the basic impact given by the most harmonious planet, which is therefore the ruler of that life. As in terrestrial music so also in the celestial there are harmonies and discords, and these all impinge upon the seed atom and aid in building the archetype. Vibratory lines of force are thus formed, which later attract and arrange physical particles as spores of sand are marshaled into geometrical figures by bowing a brass plate with a violin bow.

Along these archetypal lines of vibration the physical body is later built, and thus it expresses accurately the harmony of the spheres as it was played during the period of construction. This period, however, is much longer than the actual period of gestation, and varies according to the complexity of the structure required by the life seeking physical manifestation. Nor is the process of construction of the archetype continuous, for under aspects of the planets which produce notes to which vibratory powers of the seed atom cannot respond it simply hums over those which it has already learned, and thus engaged it waits for a new sound which it can use to build more of the organism which it desires in order to express itself.

Thus, seeing that the terrestrial organism which each of us inhabits is molded along vibratory lines produced by the song of the spheres, we may realize that the inharmonies which express themselves as disease are produced in the first place by the spiritual inharmony within. It is further evident that if we obtain accurate knowledge concerning the direct cause of the inharmony and remedy it, the physical manifestation of disease will shortly disappear. It is this information which is given by the horoscope of birth, for there each planet in its house and sign expresses harmony or discord, health or disease. Therefore, all methods of healing are adequate only in proportion as they take into consideration the stellar harmonies and discords expressed in the wheel of life--the horoscope.

While the laws of Nature that govern in the lower realms are all-powerful under ordinary circumstances, there are higher laws which pertain to the spiritual realms and which may under certain circumstances be made to supersede the former. For instance, the forgiveness of sins upon recognition thereof and true repentance is made to supersede the law which demands and eye for an eye and a tooth for a tooth. When Christ walked upon this Earth and healed the sick, He, being the lord of the Sun, embodied within Himself the synthesis of the stellar vibrations as the octave embodies all the tones of the scale, and He could therefore emit from Himself the true corrective planetary influence required in each case. He sensed the inharmony and knew at once wherewith to offset it by virtue of His exalted development. He had no need of any further preparation, but obtained results at once by substituting harmony for the planetary discord which caused the disease wherewith He was dealing. Only in one case did He take refuge in the higher law and say, "Arise, thy sins are forgiven."

Likewise with the ordinary methods employed in the Rosicrucian System of Healing, they depend upon a knowledge of the planetary inharmonies which cause disease and the correcting influence which will remedy the same. This has sufficed in all the instances which have come under our notice to date. However, there is a more powerful method available under a higher law which may accelerate recovery in cases of long standing, and under certain circumstances where the sincere and heartfelt recognition of wrong exists, may even obliterate the effects of disease before destiny, cold and hard, would otherwise so decree.

When we look with spiritual vision upon one who is diseased, whether the physical body be emaciated or not, it is plainly evident to the Seer that the finer vehicles are much more tenuous than during health. Thus they do not transmit to the physical body a proper quota of vitality, and as a consequence that instrument becomes more or less disrupted. But whatever may be the state of emaciation of the rest of the physical body, certain centers which are tenuous during health in a degree varying with the spiritual development of the man, become clogged in an increasing degree according to the seriousness of the disease. This is particularly true of the main center between the eyebrows. Therein the Spirit is immured, sometimes to such an extent that it loses touch with the outer world and its progress and becomes so thoroughly centered upon its own condition that only complete rupture of the physical body can set it free. This may be a process of long years, and in the meantime the planetary inharmony which caused the initial disease may have passed by, but the sufferer is unable to take advantage of the improved conditions. In such cases a spiritual outpouring of a special kind is necessary to bring to the soul its message, "Thy sins are forgiven." When that has been heard, it may respond to the command, "Take up thy bed and walk."

None among our present humanity can measure anywhere near the stature of the Christ, consequently none can exercise His power in such extreme cases; but the need of that power in active manifestation exists today as much as it did two thousand years ago. Spirit pervades everything in and upon our planet, but in a varying measure. It has more affinity for some substances than for others. Being an emanation from the Christ Principle, it is the Universal Spirit composing the World of Life Spirit that restores the synthetic harmony of the body.

THE LAWS OF COMPATIBILITY AND SYSTEMIC RECEPTIBILITY:

There are two basic laws in the science of Astro-therapy or healing by use of the stellar ray; one is the Law of Compatibility, the other, the law of Systemic Receptibility. By knowledge and intelligent application of these laws the sick regain health much more rapidly than otherwise and with minimum effort on the part of the health adjuster.

At the time of conception the Moon was in the degree which ascends at birth (or its opposite); the vital body was then placed in the mother's womb as a matrix into which the chemical elements forming our dense body are built. The vital body emits a sound similar to the buzz of a bumblebee. During life these etheric sound waves attract and place the chemical elements of our food so that they are formed into organs and tissues. So long as the etheric sound waves in our vital body are in harmony with the keynote of the archetype, the chemical elements wherewith we nourish our dense body are properly disposed of and assimilated, and health prevails no matter whether we are stout or thin, of rosy complexion or sallow, or whatever the outward appearance. But the moment the sound waves in the vital body vary from the archetypal key-note, this dissonance places the chemical elements of our food in a manner incongruous with the lines of force in the archetype.

Then imperfect elimination of waste, accumulation of poison in the system, and abnormal growths and other conditions become manifest in the dense body, and disease continues until harmony has been restored to the vital body. When the invisible cause has been removed, the visible effects disappear, and health is restored. Thus we see that incipient disease manifests in the vital body before the dense body begins to show signs of disability, and recovery of the vital body also precedes convalescence.

When a healthy person meets with an accident, his vital body is unimpaired; therefore he may not feel the full extent of the injury until several days afterwards. If he survives the shock of the maximum dissonance between the vital body and the archetype, the chances are good for recovery.

The pitch of the etheric vibration in the vital body is determined by the rising sign, for the reason given. Each of the twelve signs imparts a sound different from that of all the other signs, as each of the twelve signs in the chromatic scale varies from the rest. Some notes blend harmoniously and with a pleasing effect; others are basically discordant and grate upon our sensibilities. Similarly, the harmony of their rising signs makes some people agreeable and capable of helping and healing each other when necessary, while people whose rising signs are in dissonance can neither give each other help nor receive it from each other.

The first consideration, when about to undertake a case, is to discover the basic spiritual relationship between the healer and patient. If the Law of Compatibility shows harmony, the outlook is good for a speedy recovery; but where inharmony appears, the patient should be turned over to a doctor or healer with whom he is in accord.

This is the method which the Elder Brothers use in apportioning patients among Invisible Helpers, and it is the key to the success we have had in benefiting all who have applied to Headquarters for help.

Astrologically, there are four elements: Fire, Air, Earth, and Water. The planets are so many foci through which the influences of the signs are projected upon the newborn babe and give tone to the body, particularly if located in the Ascendant. The success of the healer varies in proportion as his constitution agrees with that of the patient's ascending sign, whether fiery, earthy, airy, or water.

When Saturn in the horoscope of one person occupies any degree of the zodiac included in the 1st or 6th house of another, those people are mutually incompatible and incapable of conferring benefit upon each other. Mars and Uranus also have an evil effect, but their force is quickly spent; it may be compared to the snap of a terrier. But the influence of Saturn is like the locked jaws of a bulldog, a strangle hold, a death grip, from which there is no release.

The Sun is the great reservoir of LIFE, the very opposite of Saturn; we may therefore readily see that its position would mark one as particularly beneficial to a certain class and in certain diseases. This influence is determined by its position according to triplicity. Thus, those who have the Sun in one of the fiery signs have great healing power with respect to people suffering from diseases ruled by these signs; those with the Sun in airy signs have power over diseases usual to airy signs, etc. Those born under the cardinal sign of a certain triplicity are most successful in treating acute cases of disease pertaining to those three signs; one who has the Sun in a fixed sign is apt in the cure of chronic diseases of that triplicity. Those born with the Sun in common signs make the least successful healers, but have more power to soothe the sick, and often bring recovery by their quieting influence on the patient's nerves. Therefore, they make the best nurses for patients under their triplicity, especially where there is mental trouble or where physical illness is the result of mental unrest.

Thus, people born when the Sun was in one of the fiery signs, Aries, Leo, or Sagittarius, are particularly successful in the treatment of the head, heart, spinal cord, femoral region, fevers, etc. Those born in April, with the Sun in Aries, would be best for the treatment of acute cases of those ailments. Those born in August, with the Sun in Leo, would succeed in chronic cases where others would fail, and if these healers secure a nurse having the Sun in Sagittarius, he or she will aid them in all their cases as no one else could. The same holds good of the other triplicities.

INFLUENCE OF THE MOON IN HEALING:

The Moon is the heavenly orb that brings all things to pass; whatever is foreshown by all the other planets never comes to fruition until the Moon brings it to a climax.

There is within the human body an ebb and flow, a tide, just the same as there is in the outside world. There are critical periods in certain diseases in particular that can be measured accurately by the Moon and it is therefore important that all understand the influence of this unusual planet.

There is a cosmic force that culminates at the New Moon and another at the time when the Moon is full. Everything that is started from the time of the New Moon until the full increases in intensity and finally culminates when the Moon is full. That period marks the flowing out of the life that comes from the Sun and is reflected to us by way of the Moon. This force is a great aid in building up the body and keeping it in a healthy condition. From the Full Moon to the time of the New Moon this great light force becomes darker and darker and everything that has come to a focus begins to fade and gradually dies.

Knowing that the Moon has these two influences according to whether it is increasing or decreasing, we find that in applying treatment notice must be taken of them. All treatments, like drugs, may be divided into two general classes: stimulants and sedatives. The first class has a distinctly better effect and is more easily applied during the increase of the Moon, and the other is found much more effectual if used during the Moon's decrease.

The general rule is: From the time of the New Moon to that of the Full Moon stimulants produce the greatest effect and sedatives are weakest. Decrease the dose of stimulants and increase that of sedatives. The exception is: When the Moon increasing approaches a conjunction to Saturn give larger doses of stimulants and smaller doses of sedatives.

When the Moon is increasing and approaching a conjunction to Mars and Mercury, stimulants have their maximum and sedatives their minimum effect.

When the increasing Moon is in good aspect to Jupiter and Venus cardiac stimulation produces the most lasting results. Palpitation is most effectively treated when the Moon is decreasing and aspects the before mentioned planets favorably. Apply heart stimulants with extreme care when the Moon aspects these planets unfavorably, especially when dark. Anesthetics are also then most liable to produce fatal results. If we inhibit the functioning of the pneumogastric nerve to a certain extent, we quiet the heart action and are then applying what would be the equivalent of a sedative in medicine. Manipulation of this nerve in such a way as to stimulate action is applying the equivalent of a medical stimulant.

PLANETARY POLARITIES:

When we study magnetism we are dealing with an invisible force; and ordinarily we can at best state the way it manifests in the Physical World only, as is the case whenever we deal with any FORCE. The Physical World is the world of effects; the causes are hidden from our sight, though they are nearer than hands or feet. Force is all about us, invisible and only seen by the effects it produces.

If we take a dish of water, for illustration, and allow it to freeze, we shall see a myriad of ice crystals, beautiful geometrical figures. These show the lines along which the water congealed and these lines are lines of force which were present before the water congealed; but they were invisible until the proper conditions were furnished them and they became manifest.

In the same way there are lines of force going between the two poles of a magnet; they are neither seen nor felt until we bring iron or iron filings into the place where they are, when they will manifest by arranging the filings in an orderly pattern. By making the proper conditions we may cause any of the nature forces to show their effects--moving our street cars, carrying messages with lightning speed over thousands of miles, etc., etc., but the FORCE itself is ever invisible. We know that magnetism travels always at right angles to the electric current from which it manifests; we know the difference between the manifestation of the electric and magnetic current, so dependent upon one another, but we have never seen either; though they are about the most valuable servants we have today.

Magnetism may be divided into "mineral" and "animal" magnetism, though in reality they are one, but the former has very little influence upon animal tissue, while the latter is generally impotent in working with minerals.

The mineral magnetism is derived directly from lodestones which are used to magnetize iron; this process gives to the metal thus treated the property of attracting iron. This kind of magnet is very little used, however, as its magnetism becomes depleted, is too weak in proportion to its bulk, and principally because the magnetic force cannot be controlled in such a so-called "permanent" magnet.

The "electromagnet" is also a "mineral" magnet. It is simply a piece of iron wound round with many turns of wire, and the strength of the magnet varies as the number of turns of wire, and the strength of the electric current that is passed through it.

Electricity is all about us in a diffused state, of no use for industrial purposes until it is COMPRESSED and forced through the electric wires by the powerful ELECTROMAGNETS. We must have MAGNETISM in the FIRST place before we can get any electricity. Before a new electric generator is started the "fields," which are nothing but electromagnets, must be magnetized. If this is not done they may turn it till the crack of doom, at any rate of speed they please, and it will never light a single lamp nor move a grain of weight; all depends upon the magnetism being there FIRST. After this magnetism is once started it will leave a little behind when the generator is shut down, and this so-called "residual magnetism" will be the nucleus of force to be built up each time the generator is started afresh.

All bodies of plants, animals, and men are but transformed mineral. They have all come from the mineral kingdom in the first place, and chemical analysis of the plant, animal, and human bodies brings out the fact beyond cavil. Moreover, we know that the plants get their sustenance from the mineral soil, and both animal and man are eating mineral when they consume the plants as food; even when man eats the animals he is nevertheless eating mineral compounds, and therefore he gets with his food both the mineral substances and the magnetic force which they contain.

This force we see manifesting in "hemoglobin," or the red coloring matter in the blood, which attracts the life-giving oxygen when it comes into contact with it in the millions of minute capillaries of the lungs, parting with it as readily when it passes through the capillaries which all over the body connect the arteries with the veins. Why is this?

To understand this, we must acquaint ourselves a little closer with the way magnetism manifests as seen in industrial uses.

There are always two fields or a multiple of two fields in a generator or motor, every alternate "field" or magnet being "north-pole" and every other alternating one "south-pole." If we wish to run two or more generators in "multiple" and force electricity into the same wire, the first requisite is that the magnetic current in the field-magnets should RUN IN THE SAME DIRECTION.

If that were not the case, they would not run together; they would generate currents going in OPPOSITE directions, blowing their fuses. That would be because the poles in one generator, which should have attracted, repelled, and vice versa. The remedy is to change the ends of the wire which magnetizes the field; then the magnetic current in one generator will become like the current of the other, and both will run smoothly together.

Similar conditions prevail in magnetic healing; a certain vibratory pitch and magnetic polarity were infused into each of us when the stellar forces surged through our bodies and gave us our planetary baptism at the moment when we drew our first complete breath. These are modified during our pilgrimage of life, but in the main their initial impulse remains undisturbed and therefore the horoscope at birth remains the most vital power in life to determine our sympathies and antipathies as well as all other matters. Nay, more, its pronouncements are more reliable than our conscious likes and dislikes.

Sometimes we may meet and learn to like a person, although we have a feeling that he has an inimical influence on us for which we cannot account, and therefore strive to put aside; but a comparison of his horoscope with our own will reveal the reason and if we are wise we heed its warning, or as surely as the circling stars move in their orbits around the Sun we will live to regret our disregard of this handwriting on the wall.

But there are also many cases when we do not sense the antipathy between ourselves and a certain person, though the horoscope reveals it, and if we see the signs when comparing the two horoscopes we may feel inclined to trust our feelings rather than the stellar script of the horoscopes. That also will in time lead to trouble, for the planetary polarity is certain to manifest in time unless both parties are sufficiently evolved to rule their stars in a large measure. Such people are few and far between at our present stage of evolution. Therefore we shall do well if we use our knowledge of the stellar script to compare our horoscopes with those at least who come intimately into our lives. This may save both them and us much misery and heartache. We would advise this course particularly with regard to a healer and his patients, and with reference to a prospective marriage partner.

When anyone is ill, resistance is at the lowest ebb, and on that account he is least able to withstand outside influences. So the vibrations of the healer have practically unrestrained effect, and even though he may be ensouled by the noblest of altruistic motives, desiring to pour out his very life for the benefit of the patient, if their stars were adverse at birth, his vibratory pitch and magnetism are bound to have an inimical effect upon the patient. Therefore it is of prime necessity that any healer should have a knowledge of astrology and the Law of Compatibility, whether he belongs to those who admittedly heal by magnetism and the laying on of hands or to the regular school of physicians, for the latter also infuse their vibrations into the patient's aura and help or hinder according to the agreement of their planetary polarity with that of the patient.

What has been said with regard to the healer applies with tenfold force to the nurse, for he or she is with the patient practically all the time and the contact is so much more intimate.

For healer, nurse, and patient, compatibility is determined by the rising sign, Saturn, and the 6th house. If their rising signs agree in nature so that all have fiery signs rising, or all have earthy, airy, or watery signs rising, they are harmonious, but if the patient has a watery sign rising, a nurse or a doctor with fiery signs will have a detrimental effect.

It is also necessary to see that Saturn in the horoscope of the nurse or healer is not placed in any of the degrees of the zodiac within the patient's 6th house.

CHAPTER XII

THE THERAPEUTIC BASIS OF LIGHT, COLOR, AND SOUND

God is Light.

Each time we sink ourselves in these three words we lave in a spiritual fountain of inexhaustible depth, and each succeeding time we sound more thoroughly the divine depths and draw more closely to our Father in heaven.

With every year that passes, with the aid of the greatest telescopes which the ingenuity and mechanical skill of man have been able to construct to pierce the depths of space, it becomes more evident that the infinitude of light teaches us the infinitude of God.

Truly, God is ONE and undivided. He enfolds within His being all that is, as the white light embraces all colors. But he appears threefold in manifestation, as the white light is refracted in three primary colors: blue yellow, and red. Wherever we see these colors they are emblematical of the Father, Son, and Holy Spirit. These three primary rays of divine life are diffused or radiated through the Sun and produce Life, Consciousness, and Form upon each of the seven light-bearers, the planets, which are called "the Seven Spirits before the Throne." Their names are: Mercury, Venus, Earth, Mars, Jupiter, Saturn and Uranus.

Each of the seven planets receives the light of the Sun in a different measure, according to its proximity to the central orb and the constitution of its atmosphere, and the beings upon each, according to the stage of their development have affinity for some of the solar rays. They absorb the color or colors congruous to them, and reflect the remainder upon the other planets. This reflected ray bears with it an impulse of the nature of the beings with which it has been in contact.

Thus the divine Light and Life comes to each planet, either directly from the Sun, or reflected from its six sister planets, and as the summer breeze which has wafted over blooming fields carries upon its silent invisible wings the blended fragrance of a multitude of flowers, so also the subtle influences from the garden of God bring to us the commingled impulses of all the Spirits and in that varicolored light we live and move and have our being.

The rays which come directly from the Sun are productive of spiritual illumination, the reflected rays from other planets make for added consciousness and moral development, and the rays reflected by way of the Moon give physical growth.

But as each planet can absorb only a certain quantity of one or more colors according to the general stage of evolution there, so each being upon Earth: mineral, plant, animal, and man, can absorb and thrive only upon a certain quantity of the various rays projected upon the Earth. The remainder do not affect it or produce sensation, any more than the blind are conscious of the light and color which exist everywhere around them.

The white light of the Sun contains the seven colors of the spectrum. The occultist sees even twelve colors, there being five between red and violet--going one way around the circle--in addition to the red, orange, yellow, green, etc., of the visible spectrum. Four of these colors are quite indescribable, but the fifth--the middle one of the five--is similar to the tint of a new-blown peach blossom. It is in fact the color of the vital body. Trained clairvoyants who describe it as "bluish-gray," or "reddish-gray," etc., are trying to describe a color that has no equivalent in the Physical World: and they are therefore compelled to use the nearest descriptive terms afforded by our language.

When the three primary colors are interblended, there appear four additional colors, the three secondary colors: orange, green, purple, each due to the blending of two primary colors, and one color (indigo) which contains the entire gamut of colors, making in all the seven colors of the spectrum. (Red plus yellow gives orange; blue plus yellow gives green; blue plus red gives purple.)

The color of Mars is red; of Venus, yellow; of mercury, violet; of the Moon, green; of the Sun, orange; of Jupiter, blue; of Saturn, indigo; of Uranus, yellow. We may blend these colors in order to obtain help from them. As a matter of fact, it is the complementary color which is seen in the Desire World that produces the effect of the physical colors. If it is desired to restrain one whose Mars is too prominent, the gems, colors, and metals of Saturn will help, but if we want to help someone who is moody and taciturn, we may use the gems, colors, and metals of Mars to advantage.

In the Physical World red has the tendency to excite and energize, whereas green has a cooling and a soothing effect, but the opposite is true when we look at the matter from the viewpoint of the Desire World. There the complementary color is active, and has the effect upon our desires and emotions which we ascribe to the physical color. We speak of jealousy, which is engendered by impure love, as the green-eyed monster.

Upon observing the auras of people, the trained clairvoyant notices the scarlet of anger, the gray and steel blue of fear, the darkish blue of worry, the red cloud of hate, the black veil of despair, etc. A tinge of soft sky-blue indicates hope, optimism, and a dawning religious feeling. Blue shows the highest type of spirituality, but the blue color does not appear outside the dense body save in the very greatest of saints--only yellow is usually observable there.

In the lower races the ground color of the aura is a dull red like the color of a slow burning fire, indicating their passionate, emotional nature. When we examine people upon a somewhat higher rung of the ladder of evolution, the basic color or vibration radiated by them is seen to be of an orange hue, the yellow of intellect mixed with the red of passion. The natural golden color is the Christ ray finding its chemical expression in the oxygen, a solar element, and as we advance upon the path of evolution those who are not professedly religious acquire a tinge of gold in their auras due to the higher altruistic impulses common to the West.

There is an intimate connection between color and tone; when a certain note is struck, a certain color appears simultaneously. In the heaven world color and sound are both present, but the tone is the originator of the color. Pythagoras spoke of the harmony of the spheres, and he did not use that expression simply as a poetical allusion. There is such a harmony. We are told by John that in the beginning was the Word...and without it was nothing made that was made. That was the creative fiat which first started the world into being. We hear of celestial music, for from the point of the heaven world, everything is first created in terms of sound which then molds concrete matter into the multitudinous forms which we see around us. Orderly rhythmic sound is the builder of all that is--the creator and sustainer of all form.

In the occultist's sphere of vision, the whole solar system is one vast musical instrument, spoken of in the Greek mythology as the "seven-stringed lyre of Apollo, the radiant sun god." As there are twelve semitones in the chromatic scale, so we have in the heavens, twelve signs of the zodiac, and as we have the seven keys or whole tones on the keyboard of the piano, we have seven planets. The signs of the zodiac may be said to be the sounding-board of the cosmic harp and the seven planets are the strings; they emit different sounds as they pass through the various signs, and therefore they influence mankind in diverse manner. Should the harmony fail for one single moment, should there be the slightest discord in that heavenly band, this whole universe as such must crumble. For music can destroy as well as build. This has been well proven by great musicians. For instance, the grandson of the immortal Felix Mendelssohn has for several years been experimenting with the power of sound in that direction. He has come to the conclusion that once we find the keynote of a building, bridge, or other structure, we may raze that structure to the ground by sounding that note sufficiently loud and long.

Our supercilious smiles of bygone days when listening to the story of Joshua and the walls of Jericho are no longer in place. The sound of the ram's horn undoubtedly struck the keynote of those walls which had been sensitized by the rhythmic tramp of his army in preparation for this final climax. The rhythmic tramp of many feet will destroy any bridge, and therefore soldiers are instructed to break step when crossing a bridge.

Thus we may say that every planet gives out a keynote which is the sum total of all the noises upon it, blended and harmonized by the indwelling Planetary Spirit. That sound can be heard by the Spirit ear. As Goethe says:

"The sun intones his ancient song

Mid rival chant of brother spheres;

His prescribed course he speeds along

In thunderous ways, throughout the years."

"Sound unto the spirit ear proclaims the

new-born day is here;

Rocky gates are creaking, rattling,

Phoebus' wheels are rolling, singing--

What sound intense the light is bringing."

The invisible sound-vibrations have great power over concrete matter. They both build and destroy. If a small quantity of very fine powder is placed upon a brass or glass plate, and a violin bow drawn across the edge, the vibrations will cause the powder to assume beautiful geometrical figures. The human voice is also capable of producing these figures; always the same figure for the same tone.

If one note or chord after another be sounded upon a musical instrument--a piano, or preferably a violin, for from it more gradations of tone can be obtained--a tone will finally be reached which will cause the hearer to feel a distinct vibration in the back of the lower part of the head. Each time that note is struck, the vibration will be felt. That note is the keynote of the person whom it so affects. If it be sounded in a dominant way, loud and long enough, it will kill as surely as a bullet from a pistol. If, on the other hand, it is struck slowly and soothingly it will build and rest the body, tone the nerves and restore health.

CHAPTER XIII

SLEEP AND HEALTH

THE VALUE OF SLEEP:

During the daytime the vital body specializes the colorless solar fluid which is all about us, through the organ we call the spleen. This vitality permeates the whole body and is seen by the clairvoyant as a fluid of a pale rose color, having been transmuted upon entering the physical body. It flows along every nerve, and when it is sent out by the brain centers in particularly large quantities it moves the muscles to which the nerves lead.

The vital body may be said to be built of points which stick out in all directions, inward, outward, upward, and downward, all through the body, and each little point goes through the center of one of the chemical atoms, causing it to vibrate at a higher rate than its natural speed. This vital body interpenetrates the dense body from birth till death under all conditions except when, for instance, the blood circulation stops in a certain part, as when we rest a hand upon the edge of a table for some time and it "goes to sleep," as we say. Then, if clairvoyant, we may see the etheric hand as a glove, and the chemical atoms of the hand relapse into their natural slow rate of vibration. When we slap the hand to cause it to "wake up," as we say, the peculiar prickling sensation we feel is caused by the points of the vital body which then re-enter the sleeping atoms of the hand and start them into renewed vibration.

The vital body leaves the dense body in a similar manner when a person is dying. Drowning persons who have been resuscitated experience an intense agony caused by the entrance of these points, which they feel as a prickling sensation.

During the daytime, when the solar fluid is being absorbed by the man in great quantities, these points of the vital body are blown out or distended, as it were, by the vital fluid, but as the day advances and poisons of decay clog the physical body more and more, the vital fluid flows less rapidly; in the evening there comes a time when the points in the vital body do not get a full supply of the life-giving fluid; they shrivel up and the atoms of the body move more sluggishly in consequence. Thus the Ego feels the body to be heavy, dull, and tired. At last there comes a time when, as it were, the vital body collapses and the vibrations of the dense atoms become so slow that the Ego can no longer move the body. It is forced to withdrawn in order that its vehicles may recuperate. Then we say the body has gone to sleep.

Sleep is not an inactive state, however; if it were, there would be no difference in feeling in the morning and no restorative power in sleep. The very word RESTORATION implies activity.

When a building has become dilapidated from constant wear and tear and it is necessary to renovate and restore it, the tenants move out to give the workmen full play. For similar reasons the Ego moves out of its tenement at night. As the workmen work upon the building, to make it fit for reoccupancy, so the Ego must work upon its building before it will be fit to re-enter. And such a work is done by us during the night time, although we are not conscious of it in our waking state. It is this activity which removes the poisons from the system, and as a result the body is fresh and vigorous in the morning when the Ego enters at the time of waking.

HOW TO TREAT DISEASE DURING SLEEP:

It has been asked if a person can be influenced in natural sleep as he can in hypnotic sleep, or if there is a difference. Yes, there is a difference. In the natural sleep, the Ego, clothed in the mind and desire body, draws outside the physical body and usually hovers over the body, or at any rate remains close to it, connected by the silver cord, while the vital body and the dense body are resting upon the bed.

It is then possible to influence the person by instilling into his brain the thoughts and ideas we wish to communicate. Nevertheless, we cannot then get him to do anything or to entertain any idea except that which is in line with his natural proclivities. IT IS IMPOSSIBLE TO COMMAND HIM TO DO ANYTHING AND TO ENFORCE OBEDIENCE, the same as it is when he has been driven out by the passes of the hypnotist, for it is the brain which moves the muscles, and during the natural sleep his brain is interpenetrated by his own vital body and he is in perfect control himself, while during the hypnotic sleep the passes of the hypnotist have driven the ether of which his vital body is composed out of the brain, down to the shoulders of the victim, where it lies around his neck and resembles the collar of a sweater. The dense brain is then open to the ether from the hypnotist's vital body, which displaces that of the proper owner. Thus, IN THE HYPNOTIC SLEEP THE VICTIM HAS NO CHOICE WHATEVER AS TO THE IDEAS HE ENTERTAINS OR THE MOVEMENTS HE MAKES WITH HIS BODY, but in the ordinary sleep he is still a free agent. In fact, this method of suggestion during sleep is something which mothers will find extremely beneficial in treating refractory children, for if the mother will sit by the bed of the sleeping child, hold its hand, speak to it as she would speak when it is awake, instill into its brain ideas of such a nature as she would wish it to entertain, she will find that in the waking state many of these ideas will have taken root. Also in dealing with a person who is sick or is addicted to drink, if the mother, nurse, or others use this method, they will find it possible to instill hope and healing, materially furthering recovery or aiding self-mastery.

THE EFFECT OF HYPNOTIC SLEEP:

From the occult viewpoint it is obviously wrong to try to cure a bad habit, such as drunkenness, by hypnotism. Looked at from the standpoint of one life, such methods as those employed by the healers of the Immanuel Movement, etc., are undoubtedly productive of an immense amount of good. The patient is seated in a chair, put into sleep and there he is given certain so-called "suggestions." He rises and is cured of his bad habit; from being a drunkard he becomes a respectable citizen who cares for his wife and family, and upon the face of it the good seems to be undeniable.

But looking at it from the deeper standpoint of the occultist, WHO VIEWS THIS LIFE AS ONLY ONE IN MANY, and looking at it from the effect is has upon the invisible vehicles of man, the case is vastly different. When a man is put into a hypnotic sleep, the hypnotist makes passes over him which have the effect of expelling the ether from the head of his dense body and substituting the ether of the hypnotist. The man is then under the perfect domination of another; he has no free will, and, therefore, the so- called "suggestions" are in reality COMMANDS which the victim has no choice but to obey. Besides, when the hypnotist withdraws his ether and wakens the victim he is unable to remove all the ether he put into him. To use a simile, as a small part of the magnetism infused into an electric dynamo before it can be started for the first time is left behind and remains as residual magnetism to excite the fields of the dynamo every time it is started up, so also there remains a small part of the ether of the hypnotist's vital body in the medulla oblongata of the victim, which is a club the hypnotist holds over him all his life, and it is due to this fact that suggestions to be carried out at a period subsequent to the awakening of the victim are invariably followed.

Thus the victim of a hypnotic healer does not overcome the bad habit by his own strength, but is as much chained in that respect as if he were in solitary confinement, and although in this life he may seem to be a better citizen, when he returns to Earth in another embodiment he will have the same weakness and have to struggle until at last he overcomes it himself.

PROTECTIVE INFLUENCE:

There are methods of protecting oneself from inimical influences, and it is better to be enlightened concerning things that threaten so that we may take whatever precautions are necessary to meet the emergency.

When we live lives of purity, when our days are filled with service to God and to our fellow men, and with thoughts and actions of the highest nobility, then we create for ourselves the GOLDEN WEDDING GARMENT, which is a radiant force for good. No evil is able to penetrate this armor, for the evil acts as a boomerang and recoils on the one who sent it, bringing to him the evil he wished others.

It is a fact than an auric atmosphere surrounds every human being. We know that often we feel the presence of a person whom we do not see, and we feel it because there is this atmosphere outside of our dense bodies. This is gradually changing; gradually it is becoming more and more golden in the West. The farther we go with the Sun, the more this golden color increases--the color of the Christ and of the Christ-like, the saints whom painters have depicted with a halo.

Gradually we are becoming more like Him, and this SOMA PSUCHICON or soul body is taking shape, is being made ready as our "Wedding Garment."

But, alas, none of us are altogether good. We know only too well the war between the flesh and the Spirit. We cannot hide from ourselves the fact that like Paul, "the good that we would do, we do not, and the evil that we would shun, that we do." Far too often our good resolutions come to naught and we do wrong because it is easier. Therefore, we all have the nucleus of evil within ourselves, which affords the open sesame for evil forces to work upon. For that reason it is best for us not to expose ourselves unnecessarily at places where seances are held with Spirits invisible to us, no matter how fine their teachings may sound to the unsophisticated. Neither should we take part even as spectators at hypnotic demonstrations, for there also a negative attitude lays one liable to the danger of obsession. We should at all times follow the advice of Paul and put on the whole armor of God. We should be positive in our fight for the good against the evil and never let an occasion slip to aid the Elder Brothers by word or deed in the Great War for spiritual supremacy.

CHAPTER XIV

MIND AND HEALING

THE TRUE CAUSE OF CONTAGION:

There are many people of a supercilious nature who are always ready to crack a joke at the expense of those who practice methods of divine healing which teach one to cultivate a fearless attitude of mind under all conditions. But as a matter of actual fact, an enormous percentage of our sickness is actually due and traceable to feelings of fear upon the part of the patient.

Travelers who have visited uninhabited islands report that the birds and beasts found there were unafraid of them at first, but they soon learned the predatory nature of man and fled before him in fear of their lives. thus the ruthless nature of man has in ages past, spread fear all over the Earth. We have conquered, tamed and exploited both bird and beast, and what we could not conquer we have slain, until every breathing thing hides in fear of us. That is to say, among the larger animals--none is so large that it does not fear us and flee from us.

When we turn in the direction of the little things then the case is different. Man, who thinks he reigns supreme on Earth because he has put all the larger creation in a state of fear, trembles in turn before the minute things in the world and the smaller they are, the more he fears them. The microscope has told us that such a small creature as the housefly carries about on the fur of its legs thousands of parasites, and therefore fear prompts us to spend millions of dollars on fly-paper, fly-screens, flytraps, and other devices to rid ourselves of this pest, but our efforts are largely in vain. Though vast sums are expended yearly to exterminate the fly, it is so prolific that is breeds faster than we can slay.

We fear its cousin, the mosquito, even more. The microscope has told us that this little insect is one of the chief messengers of the Angel of Death. Therefore we fight it in fear of our lives, but it thrives in spite of the vast sums yearly expended upon its termination. Then there is the milk we drink. Under ordinary conditions it is said that there are 100,000 germs to the cubic centimeter, but under the best and most sanitary conditions this army of destroyers can be brought down to 10,000. So in fear and trembling we pasteurize this fluid before we dare to give it to the children of tender age. Every drop of water we drink swarms with germ life, says the microscope, and even the coin and currency wherewith we purchase the necessities of life are vehicles of death, for they are infected with germs to an almost unbelievable extent. Once we started to launder them, but it was found that the bankers could not so easily detect counterfeits after they had been washed, so we abandoned the process. We either fear the counterfeiters more than the germs or we love money more than health.

Is not this whole attitude ridiculous and unworthy of our high and noble estate, as human beings, as children of God? It is well known to science that an attitude of fear breaks down the power of resistance of the body, and thereby lays it liable to diseases which would not otherwise be able to gain a foothold. From the occult point of view it is perfectly plain why this is so. The dense body which we see with our eyes it interpenetrated by a vehicle made of ether, and the energy from the Sun, which pervades all space, is constantly pouring into our body through the spleen which is a specialized organ for the attraction and assimilation of this universal ether. In the solar plexus it is converted into a rose colored fluid which permeates the nervous system.

This may be compared to electricity in the wires of an electric or telegraphic system. By means of this vital fluid the muscles are moved and the organs perform their vital functions so that the body may express itself in perfect health. The better the health the larger the quantity of this solar fluid which we are able to absorb, but we only utilize a certain part of it and the surplus is radiated from the body in straight lines.

You have seen the paper ribbons fastened in front of electric fans in candy stores and fruit stands. When the fan is set going these streamers float outwards from the fan. The streamers which flow from the whole periphery of the human body also radiate in straight lines when we are in perfect health. This condition is therefore aptly described as radiant health. We speak of such a person as radiating life and vigor. Under such conditions no disease germs can ever get a foothold in his body. They cannot enter from without because of these invisible streamers of force, any more than a fly an enter an opening in a building covered by an exhaust fan. And those microorganisms which enter the body with the food are also quickly expelled, for the vital processes in the body are selective as shown by the kidneys, for instance, which excrete the waste matter while retaining vital substances necessary for the economy of the body.

But the moment we allow thoughts of fear, of worry, of anger, the body endeavors, as it were, to close the gates against an outside foe, fancied or real. Then also the spleen closes up and ceases to specialize the vital fluid in sufficient quantities for the necessities of the body, and we then see a phenomenon which is analogous to the effect of lowering the voltage or cutting in more resistance in the electric fan. In that case the paper streamers will begin to hang down, they will no longer wave over the candy or fruit to protect it and keep the flies away. Similarly in the human body, when the thought of fear forces the partial closure of the spleen, the solar fluid does not go through the body with the same speed as before. It does not then radiate from the periphery in straight lines, but these lines become crumpled and thus they allow easy access to the little deleterious organisms which may then feed unobstructed upon our tissues and cause disease.

Whether the consistent mental scientists, or others who believe in divine healing, know this law or not, they act according to its dictates when they affirm that they are children of God, that they have no reason to fear, for God is their Father and will protect them so long as they do not deliberately disregard the ordinary laws of life.

The actual fact, and the truth in the matter is that contagion comes from within. So long as we live a common-sense life, feeding our bodies upon the pure foods which come from the vegetable kingdom, taking a sufficient amount of exercise, and keeping mentally active, we may rest secure in the promise that the Lord is our refuge. There shall no evil befall us so long as we thus show our faith by our works. On the other hand, if we belie our faith in God by disregard of His laws our expectations of health are vain.

POWER OF THOUGHT:

"As a man thinketh in his heart so is he," said the Christ, and this is an absolutely scientific proposition; something, moreover, which everyone may demonstrate by looking about him in the everyday conditions of life in the home, office, or street. Here we see a man with thick lips, with puffed cheeks, with a veritable pouch under his chin, and at once we know that we have before us a glutton and a sensualist. Another comes along the street; his face is furrowed by lines, his lips are thin and set, and we know that thought and care have been the architects that molded his face.

Each one who passes expresses without exactly what his thoughts are within. One is muscular and active, because the thoughts which have governed his activities built an active body. Another has flabby flesh, a pouch stomach, and a waddling walk, showing that he is averse to all exercise. In each case the body is an accurate reproduction of the mind; each class suffers from the ailments peculiar to the trend of its mental activity. The glutton and sensualist suffer from diseases engendered when their thoughts have crystallized and weakened the digestive tract and creative organs. Their diseases are entirely different from the nervous diseases that attack the thinker, and any system of healing that does not take into consideration the fact that the body is more a physical expression of mind than mind is a manifestation of the physical man, makes a very radical mistake. In our complex nature, mind and matter act and react upon each other in such a manner that it is absolutely necessary to consider the man as a whole whenever we attempt to deal with his disability.

It is well known to physiologists that joy will sometimes bring the patient out of the sick room quicker than any medicine. If something has happened to give his affairs in the world a sudden upward turn, so that he becomes optimistic, disease seems to disappear as if by magic; and conversely, even though he may seem to enjoy good health, the moment a depressing influence comes into his business affairs he begins to feel ill in body. A letter containing bad news may sometimes stop direction entirely, and give the person who receives it a very serious attack of indigestion. Thus the truth of the Savior's teaching that "As a man thinketh in his heart, so is he," is amply demonstrated in practical, everyday life.

When we realize this we also see the necessity of cultivating an attitude of optimism. A hopeful mind is the greatest of all medicine, and a constant reiteration of a resolution to overcome the present ills, is better than all the medicine in the world. When one is in constant pain, suffering acutely, it is perhaps very difficult to maintain an attitude of optimism, nevertheless, the magic formula of the Savior applied to health, will help us to overcome in time.

It is a law that if we think health we must of necessity sooner or later express health. We must live the rational life and cease from excesses, particularly in diet; that cannot be emphasized too often. Neither, will it avail to stand before a mirror and reiterate to oneself, "I have Faith," "I am Health," or similar untrue affirmations. Just stop talking of your ailments to others; try above all to divert your own thoughts from your condition; believe in health as our birthright, and as something that can be attained by us, never wavering.

You may have heard the story of the old lady who had heard her minister speak about a faith that could remove mountains. She was willing to try her faith on the ash heap, but next morning when she saw it was still there she exclaimed, "I thought so." Conditions were what she expected in her heart, not what she claimed to believe with her tongue, and it will be the same with everyone. Therefore, believe heartily in health.

CHAPTER XV

DANGERS OF EXCESSIVE BATHING

While cleanliness itself is a virtue, it becomes, like many another good thing, a vice by being overdone. Water is the universal solvent and taken internally in small doses it is good, but taken at the wrong time, with meals for instance, and in excess, it becomes a poison. It dilutes the digestive fluids and cools the stomach so that the condition necessary for the proper treatment of the food is disarranged and in time, if the habit is persisted in, it impairs the digestion permanently. So also when water is taken in excess outside and under improper conditions, it may affect the health very seriously.

This has been demonstrated many times in our experiences on Mt. Ecclesia. A number of people who came here have been in the habit, prior to their arrival, of bathing every day and sometimes twice or three times a day. They were, without exception, in a very serious run-down condition, because the excess of water applied with a towel or a sponge, had depleted the skin of its fatty substance, and the vasomotor system was unable to operate properly, to close or open the pores as required.

But there was another effect of this excessive bathing, not seen or understood unless by one who has the requisite occult knowledge, and the spiritual sight to investigate the matter properly. Others may know the truth of the following explanation because of their own experience along the lines of healing and magnetism.

We all know that when we take a physician's galvanic battery and place one electrode in a basin of water, holding the other electrode in the hand, the flow of electricity through the body is much stronger than when we put our other hand in the water or if we hold both electrodes without contact with water. When water is evaporated its molecules are broken up and each fragment is then enclosed in an envelope of ether which will act as a cushion and is the basis of elasticity in steam. When condensation takes place the surplus of ether disappears, and water becomes incompressible as the solid rock.

But water has great yearning for ether; it cannot take it from the air, however, any more than we can absorb nitrogen though we breathe it continually. Fluid is volatile in proportion to the amount of ether it contains, and we have an example of the intense greed of water for ether in the avidity wherewith it absorbs anhydrous ammonia, a fluid so volatile that it boils at 26 degrees below zero. This shows why water causes so voluminous a flow between a battery electrode and the body, and explains many phenomena, among others, why moisture aids so materially in transmitting good magnetism, the vital fluid of the healer to his patient, and withdrawing bad magnetism from the body of the latter. Also how necessary and helpful it is to wash in running water, so that the poisonous ether taken out of the patient's vital body will not hamper the healer. When we take a bath under ordinary normal circumstances, we remove a great deal of effete poisonous ether from our vital bodies provided we stay in a reasonable length of time. After a bath the vital body becomes somewhat attenuated and consequently gives us a feeling of weakness, but if we are in ordinary good health and have not stayed in the bath too long, the deficiency is soon made good by the stream of force which flows into the human body through the spleen. When this recuperation has taken place we feel renewed vitality and attribute it to the bath without realizing THE FULL FACTS as above stated.

But when a person who is not in perfect health commences to bathe every day, perhaps twice or three times a day, an excess of ether is taken from the vital body. The new supply entering by way of the spleen is also diminished on account of the attenuated condition of the vital body; thus it is impossible for such persons to recuperate after repeated depletions and as a consequence the health of the dense body suffers; they lose almost every ounce of strength and gradually become confirmed invalids. Being in this delicate state they are unable to eat and assimilate truly nourishing foods and in time their condition may become very, very serious.

Cases of this description are exceedingly difficult to handle, because they usually occur with people with common signs on the angles, with many planets in these signs, or with the Sun or Ascendant there. This class of people resent any interference with their diet and habit of bathing, because they think they are paragons of cleanliness, which is in their eyes a chief virtue. They believe they cannot live without so many baths daily and as their appetite is so slight and delicate they believe that they know better than anyone else how to look after that part of their requirements, but they are wrong in both cases as shown in the foregoing.

Their first step to health involves that they cease bathing entirely. The dry bath is the proper restorative, and for this purpose a pair of coarse gloves made of linen tape loosely woven are best. With these the body may be rubbed morning and evening until the skin shows a health glow. By this process the superfluous cuticle is removed but the oil and ether remain. Thus the patient will build up very rapidly, for when the chemical ether increases, the power of assimilation also revives and there is an immediate gain of both strength and flesh. If necessary the patient may be given a very light warm sponge bath once a week, but no tub baths should be attempted until he or she is fully recovered.

CHAPTER XVI

TRANSFUSION OF BLOOD

Among the latest discoveries of science is haemolysis--the fact that inoculation of blood from the veins of a higher animal into one of a lower species, destroys the blood of the lower animal and causes its death. Thus the blood of man injected into the veins of any animal is fatal. But from man to man it is found that transfusion may take place, although at times there are deleterious effects.

In olden days people married in the family; it was then looked upon with horror if one should "seek after strange flesh." When the sons of God married the daughters of men, that is to say, when the subjects of one leader married outside the tribe, there was great trouble, they were cast off by their leader and destroyed, for at that time certain qualities that we now possess were to be developed in humanity and were thus implanted in the common blood which ran pure in the family or small tribe. Later on when man was to be brought down into material conditions, international marriages were commanded, and, from that time on, it has been looked upon as equally horrible if persons within the same family united in marriage.

The old Vikings would not allow anyone to marry into their family unless they had first gone through the ceremony of mixing blood to see if the transfusion of the blood of the stranger into their family was detrimental or otherwise. All this was because in earlier times humanity was not as individualized as it is today. They were more under the domination of the Race or Family Spirit, which dwelt in their blood, as the Group Spirit of animals does in the blood of animals. Later the international marriages were given to free humanity from that yoke and make every separate Ego sole master of its own body without outside interference.

Science has lately found that the blood of different people has different crystals, so that it is possible now to tell the blood of a Negro from the blood of a white man; but there will come a day when they will know a still greater difference, for just as there is a difference in the crystals formed by the different races, so there is also a difference in the crystals formed by each individual man. The thumb-marks of no two people are alike, and it will be found in time that the blood of each human being is different from the blood of every other individual. This difference is already evident to the occult investigator, and it is only a question of time when science will make the discovery, for the distinguishing features are becoming more marked as the human being grows less and less dependent, more and more self-sufficient.

This change in the blood is most important and in time, when it has become more marked, it will be productive of most far-reaching consequences. It is said that "Nature geometrizes," and Nature is but the visible symbol of the invisible God whose offspring and images we are. Being made in His likeness, we are also beginning to geometrize, and naturally we are starting on the substance where we, the human spirits, the Egos, have the greatest power, namely, in our blood.

When the blood comes through the arteries, which are deep in the body, it is a gas; but loss of heat nearer the surface of the body causes it to partially condense, and in that substance the Ego is learning to form mineral crystals. In the Jupiter Period we shall learn to invest them with a low form of vitality and set them out from ourselves as plant-like structures. In the Venus Period we shall be able to infuse desire into them and make them like animals. Finally, in the Vulcan Period, we shall give them a mind and rule over them as race spirits.

At the present time we are at the very beginning of this individualization of our blood. Therefore it is possible at present to transfuse blood from one human being to another, but the day is near at hand when that will be impossible. The blood of a white man will kill all who stand lower, and the blood of an advanced person will poison the less cultured. The child at present receives its supply of blood from the parents, stored in the thymus gland, for the years of childhood. But the time will come when the Ego will be too far individualized to function in blood not generated by itself. Then the present mode of generation will have to be superseded by another whereby the Ego may create its own vehicle without the help of parents.

CHAPTER XVII

EFFECTS OF REMOVAL OF PHYSICAL ORGAN

Generally speaking, when an arm, a limb, or an organ has been removed from the physical body by means of a surgical operation, the dense part of the organ permeated by the planetary ether is taken away. The four ethers which constitute the vital body of the man or woman thus operated upon remain; but there is a certain magnetic connection between the part decaying in the grave and that etheric counterpart which remains with the person. Therefore, he or she feels the pain and suffering in the part removed for some time after an operation, until decay has taken place and the etheric counterpart has disintegrated.

However, there are some exceptions to this general rule which it is well to note. We have observed that the physical body accommodates itself so far as possible to altered conditions. If a wound in a certain part of the body makes it impossible for the blood to flow in the normal channels it finds another set of veins by which it may make its circuit, but an organ never atrophies so long as it can serve any useful purpose. It is similar with the vital body composed of ethers. When an arm or limb has been amputated, the etheric counterpart of that member is no longer required in the economy of the body; therefore, it gradually wastes away. But in the case of an organ like the spleen where the etheric counterpart has an important function as gateway for the solar energy, naturally no such disintegration will take place.

It should also be remembered that wherever disease manifests in the physical vehicle that part of the vital body has first become thin, attenuated, and diseased, and it was its failure to supply the necessary vital energy that caused the manifestation of physical symptoms of ill health. Conversely, when health returns, the vital body is the first to pick up, and this convalescence is then manifested in the dense body. Therefore, if the physical spleen is diseased, it is a foregone conclusion that the etheric counterpart is also in subnormal health, and the wisdom of removing the organ is doubtful. However, if it is done, the body will seek to accommodate itself to the new condition and the etheric counterpart of the spleen will continue to function as before.

Another interesting angle to this question is revealed in the after-death state. When a person who is injured passes into the invisible realm, he thinks with the same mind, pictures himself there as he was in the world. Consequently a scar on the forehead or the loss of an arm or limb is reproduced by his thought in the matter of the Desire World, and he appears there disfigured as he was here. In the World War this was very noticeable, for all the soldiers who passed out with wounds which they could see and which they knew how to determine the effect of, reproduced these wounds in their desire bodies. They felt pain similar to what they would have felt if they had still been in the physical body, because they fancied that there must be pain connected with it. However, they were quickly assisted by one another and by those who had been helped by the Elder Brothers to see the matter right: that there was no actual pain. As soon as they were convinced that their wounds were but illusions and taught that they could shape their bodies in the normal and healthy state, they could quickly remedy the condition.

REMOVAL OF TONSILS:

Removal of the tonsils is a subject on which our opinion is frequently asked, and we have always discouraged the removal of these necessary organs, for it has been found that serious throat and lung diseases are often experienced in later life as a consequence of removing the tonsils, and an increasing number of physicians today denounce this operation as wholly unnecessary.

The tonsils are ruled by Taurus, one of the signs of Venus. There is great sympathy between signs ruled by the same planet. Libra, the other Venus sign, rules the kidneys. Removal of tonsils from the Taurus region affects secretion of urine in the Libra region. Therefore, when we remove the tonsils from a child we increase the tendency to gout and rheumatism in later years.

As a matter of fact, enlarged tonsils are due to conditions connected with the arrival at puberty and adolescence, perhaps accentuated by a wrong diet, and this is a factor in most of the other throat diseases, for the larynx is the opposite of the generative organs, as proved by the fact that the voice changes at the time of puberty; and in many other ways. When the period of adolescence is past it will be found that these organs will return to their normal condition and will give no further trouble.

In acute conditions we have always recommended the citrus fruits as the finest antiseptics known. This applies also and particularly to pineapple. Lemonade made of lemons and HONEY will be found to give great relief in this condition. Oranges, grapefruit, and pineapple should also be used freely when the child complains of throat trouble. A cold compress on the throat at night when the child goes to bed, supplemented by massage of the throat, will be found an effective treatment in all throat troubles. It goes without saying that the bowels should be kept open and clear. By the use of these simple treatments the trouble will probably be over in a few days, perhaps even without the necessity of putting the child to bed. Do not be afraid if white matter is expectorated during the process of this treatment. That is just what the child needs to get rid of, in order to be well.

CHAPTER XVIII

FORM OF HEALING TO USE

INTRODUCTION:

The form of healing to advise depends upon the nature of the sickness and the temperament of the patient. If it is a case of a broken leg, a surgeon is obviously the one to call. If there is an internal disorder and it is possible to get a broad-minded physician, then in certain cases he is the one to get. If, on the other hand, a mental healer, Christian Science healer, or anyone else who is spiritually minded can be brought in, HE MAY HELP A PERSON WHO IS HIMSELF STRONG IN FAITH, for, as a tuning fork which is of a certain pitch will respond when another tuning fork of the same pitch is struck, so will the person filled with faith respond to the ministrations of these last named ones. But where faith in their methods is lacking in the patient, it is far better to send for a regular physician in whom the patient has confidence, for health or sickness depends almost altogether upon the state of mind, and in the conditions of sickness where a person is enfeebled, he becomes hypersensitive and should not be thwarted in his preferences. Besides, whatever good there is in any system of healing, the effects upon a certain person will be beneficial or the reverse in exact proportion to his faith in its healing power.

TAKING MEDICINE:

Certainly, it is our duty to take medicine administered by a properly qualified person, or attempt to cure the ills from which we suffer in any other way possible that appeals to us. We should be doing decidedly wrong if we allowed our physical instrument to deteriorate for lack of proper care and attention. It is the most valuable tool we possess, and unless we use it circumspectly and care for it, we are amenable to the Law of Cause and Effect for that neglect.

LAYING ON OF HANDS:

There are two very common difficulties in the practice of osteopathy and kindred methods of treatment by the laying on of hands. In this process there are two distinct operations. One is a taking away from the patient of something that is poisonous and injurious, provocative of disease; and there is also a giving out of vital force by the doctor himself, or herself. Everybody who had done any work of this kind knows this because it has been felt and is felt by every one who is successful. Now, unless the doctor or healer is bubbling over with radiant health, two things are liable to happen; either the human miasma taken away from the patient may so overwhelm him or her that to use a common expression "he takes on the condition" of the patient, or he may give too much of his own vital force, and thus become entirely depleted. Both of these conditions may combine, and then there comes a day when the physician or healer finds himself or herself run down and forced to rest.

Magnetic healers who are frankly unscientific often escape the first-mentioned condition by "throwing off the magnetism," as they say, but all are liable to be run down. That is something that nobody can escape, save on who can see the etheric effluvia he takes and the vital fluid he gives. Most people are vampires when they are sick, and the stronger and more robust they are ordinarily, the worse they are usually when sickness has thrown them upon a bed or sickness.

The following hint is of value in keeping away undesirable conditions: First, fix your thoughts firmly in such a manner that you will not allow this miasmatic effluvia which leaves the patient's body to enter your body further than the elbow; second, when you are giving treatment leave the patient once in a while and wash your hands IN RUNNING WATER IF POSSIBLE; but at any rate wash in water, and change the water as frequently as possible. The water has a twofold effect. In the first place, the effluvia leaving the patient's body has an affinity for water. In the second place, the moisture which stays upon your hands enables you to get the miasma from the patient in a larger measure than you otherwise would. This is on the very same principle that if you take the electrodes of an electrical battery and put them into water, you will find the effect of electricity is many times intensified if you try to touch the water.

So also with yourself; you are the electric battery in the case, and your hands being moistened will draw to yourself the miasma in a much greater measure than otherwise. If conditions are such that you cannot get water you may try to throw the magnetism off, but then it is necessary to be careful, because when the magnetism is thrown away from you it is attracted to the Earth, because it is subject to gravity; and to the spiritual vision it is a dark or rather a black jelly-like fluid. It lies shimmering and shivering on the floor. If now the patients gets up relieved from the couch where treatment has been given, and goes over the place where this magnetism has been thrown away, then the miasma will re-enter the body and he or she will be in a worse condition than before you started the treatment. Therefore it is the best policy always to throw such miasma our of the window, or better still, put them into a fireplace and then set fire to them.

From the foregoing it is evident that this laying on of hands is something that should not be done indiscriminately by any one who has not been trained in one of the many properly equipped schools of Osteopathy, Chiropractic, etc. Probationers who live worthy lives are trained under the special guidance of the Elder Brothers.

VACCINATION AND ANTITOXIN:

Bacteriologists have discovered that many diseases are caused by microorganisms which invade our body, and also that when this invading army begins to create a disturbance the body commences to manufacture germs of an opposing nature or a substance which will poison the invaders. It is them a question of which are the strongest, the invaders or the defenders. If the defending microbes are more numerous than the invaders or if the poison which is noxious to the invaders is manufactured in sufficient quantities, the patient recovers. If the defenders are vanquished on the body is unable to manufacture a sufficient quantity of the serum necessary to poison the invaders, the patient succumbs to the disease. It was further discovered than when a certain person has once successfully recovered from a specific malady, he is immune from renewed attacks of that disease for the reason that he has in his body the serum which is death to the germs that cause the disease he has once weathered.

From the above facts certain conclusions were drawn:

(1) If a healthy person is inoculated with a few of the germs of a certain disease he will contract that disease in a mild form. He will then be able to develop the saving serum and thus he will become immune to that disease in the future.

THAT IS THE PHILOSOPHY OF VACCINATION AS A MEANS OF PREVENTING DISEASE.

(2) When a person has contracted a disease and is unable to manufacture a sufficient quantity of the serum which will destroy the invading microorganisms, his life may be saved by inoculation with the serum obtained from another who has become immune.

As it is not easy to get such antitoxins or cultures from human beings, these germ-cultures and poisons have been obtained from animals, and much has been written both for and against the use of such methods of fighting disease. With these we are not here concerned; the occult viewpoint goes deeper than the question at issue, as seen from the material side of life. There are undoubtedly cases where disease has been prevented by the use of antitoxin; there are also cases where vaccination and antitoxin have caused the fatality they were designed to prevent, but that is beside the question. From the occult viewpoint vaccination and the use of antitoxin OBTAINED BY THE PROCESSES IN USE IN BACTERIOLOGICAL INSTITUTES is to be deplored. These methods work a wrong on the helpless animals and POISON THE HUMAN BODY, making it difficult for the Ego to use its instrument.

If we study the chemistry of our food we shall find that nature has provided all necessary medicine, and if we eat right we shall be immune from disease without vaccination.

When in normal health the body specializes a far greater quantity of the solar energy than it can use. The surplus is radiated form the whole surface of the body with great force and prevents the entrance of microorganisms which lack the strength to battle against the outwelling current; nay, more! on the same principle that an exhaust fan will gather up particles of dust in a room and hurl them outward does this vital fluid cleanse the body of inimical matter, dangerous germs included., It must not surprise us that this force is intelligent and capable of selecting the materials which should be eliminated, leaving the beneficial and useful. Scientist recognize this fact of selective osmosis. They know that while a sieve will allow any particle of matter to pass through which is smaller than the mesh of the sieve, the kidneys for instance, will keep fluids of use to the body, while allowing waste products to pass. In as similar manner the vital fluid makes a distinction, it rids the body of the poisons and impurities generated inside and repels similar products from without.

This emanation has been called N-rays, or Odic fluid, by scientist who have discovered it by means of chemical reagents which render it luminous. During the process of digestion it is weakest, for then an extra quantity of the solar energy is required for use inside the body in the metabolism of the food; it is the cementing factor in assimilation. The heartier we have eaten, the greater is the quantity of vital fluid expended WITHIN THE BODY and the weaker the eliminative and protecting outrushing current. Consequently we are in the greatest danger from an invasion by an army of inimical microorganisms when we have gorged ourselves.

On the other hand, if we eat sparingly and choose the foods which are the most easily digestible, the diminution of the protective vital current will be correspondingly minimized and our immunity from disease will be much enhanced without the necessity of poisoning our body with vaccine.

CHAPTER XIX

THE SCOPE OF HEALING

THE LAW OF DESTINY:

A large and increasing number of medical men are now convinced that the LAW OF DESTINY is an important factor in producing disease and retarding recovery, though they are not believers in the fallacy of an inexorable fate. They recognize that God DOES NOT WILLINGLY AFFLICT US NOR AIM TO GET EVEN WITH THE TRANSGRESSOR; they understand that all sorrow and suffering are designed to teach us lessons which we would not or could not learn in any other way. The stars show the period estimated as requisite to teach us the lesson; but EVEN GOD CANNOT DETERMINE THE EXACT TIME nor the amount of suffering necessary; we, ourselves, have a prerogative, FOR WE ARE DIVINE. If we awake to our transgression and commence to obey the law ere the stellar affliction ceases, we are cured of our mental, moral, or physical distemper; if we persist to the end of one stellar affliction without having learned our lesson, a more inimical configuration will enforce obedience at a later time.

Cancer and consumption are seemingly incurable, yet there is always a possibility that they may yield, and they certainly will yield, if the force directed against them is sufficient. Like all other physical manifestation, they are the result of a spiritual cause, and if we can get at that, offset it with something of an opposite nature, there is a chance, whereas the attitude of resignation and non-assistance will certainly never bring the patient out of his or her condition. Given life in a salubrious climate--a strong desire for health, a hope that neither knows or permits of discouragement--and a simple, nutritious, healthful diet will cure even the worst case of consumption. As for cancer, it is difficult to tell when the debt of destiny which has caused the trouble has passed, and there are many cases on record where cancer has been cured; that is to say, of course, in its milder forms; but even in its advanced forms there is no reason for giving up hope as long as there is life.

As for sclerosis, there are several methods whereby the deposits may be eliminated, and these removed, the patient may become as well as ever. Particularly is this so if he or she can be brought to recognize the breach of the laws of Nature which has caused the disease in the specific case, and it is to this end that we should labor. Whether the disease be cured or not, if the person can be taught now what laws have been transgressed, if he or she can be led to see what is the spiritual cause of the disease, and learn to walk in the ways of virtue, which are according to the laws of God, then in the future there will be no disease for them. It is that for which we are laboring, that we may hasten the day of liberation; that we may bring all mankind towards a realization of health.

As to whether or not we should interfere with destiny, let us first realize who made the destiny! We did! We set the force going which has now ripened into destiny, and having made it, we certainly have the right to change it in so far as we are able. In fact, this is the hall mark of divinity, to rule ourselves. The very greatest majority of mankind is ruled by the heavenly orbs which may be called "the clock of destiny." The twelve signs of the zodiac mark the twelve hours of day and night, the planets may be likened to the hour hand and show the year when a certain debt of destiny is ripe for expression in our life. The Moon indicates the month, and attracts certain influences felt by us without our knowing that they are being exerted, or without our realizing what they are for, but these influences will tend to bring our actions in line with the destiny which we have made in previous lives, and invariably the thing which is foreshown will come to pass unless--yes, there is an UNLESS, thank God, for if it were not so, if there were no possibility of changing destiny, then let us sit down, "Let us eat, drink, and be merry, for tomorrow we die." We should then be in the hands of inexorable fate and unable to help ourselves. But, thank God there is one chance which is not shown in the horoscope, namely, that the human will may assert itself and frustrate fate.

As Ella Wheeler Wilcox has expressed in poetic form:

"One ship sails east and another sails west,

With the selfsame winds that blow.

'Tis the set of the sail, and not the gale

Which determines the way they go."

It is of utmost importance that we set the sails of the barque of life as we want and never scruple about interfering with fate.

This disposes also of the idea of "affirmation" as a factor in life. This in itself is folly. It is work and action that we need in life, as you will readily see by this illustration. Suppose a little seed of those beautiful carnations were endowed with speech, and it came to you saying: "I am a carnation." Would you not answer: "No, you are not a carnation, you foolish little thing. You have the potentiality in you, but you will have to go out in the garden and bury yourself for awhile and grow. By that process alone you can become a carnation, never by affirmation." Similarly with ourselves. All the "affirmations" of divinity are vain unless accompanies by actions of a divine character, and they will prove our divinity as words never can.

RELATION TO SPIRITUALITY TO HEALTH:

The rupture of physically robust health is necessary before it is possible to attain poise in the spiritual world, and the stronger and more vigorous the instrument, the more drastic must be the method of breaking it down. Then come years when there is an unbalanced fluctuating condition of health, until finally we are able to adjust ourselves so as to maintain health in the Physical World while we retain the ability to function also in the higher realms.

When we understand the higher philosophies, when we live the life that is taught by them, our body becomes extremely sensitive and must be given more care than is necessary to the body of an Indian, or Negro in the wilds of Africa. They have no delicately organized nervous system like the white race. Those who are interested along the lines of spiritual development are particularly high-strung, therefore, as we progress it becomes necessary to take more and more care of this instrument. But we also learn the laws of its nature and how to conform to them. If we apply our knowledge it is possible for us to have a sensitive instrument and keep it in comparative health.

There are cases, however, when a sickness is necessary to bring about certain changes in the body which are the precursors of a higher step in spiritual unfoldment, and under such conditions, of course, sickness is a blessing and not a curse. In general, however, it may be said that the study of the higher philosophy will always tend to better one's health, because "knowledge is power" and the more we know the better we are able to cope with all conditions, provided, of course, we bring our knowledge into practice and LIVE THE LIFE--that we are not merely hearers of the word, but doers also, for no teaching is of benefit to us unless it is carried into our lives and lived from day to day.

NERVOUSNESS HELPED BY EXERCISES:

If a person of a nervous temperament will endeavor to perform calmly and quietly the exercises of Retrospection and Concentration, he will experience a very beneficial effect, particularly if he will strive to RELAX EVERY MUSCLE of the body during the exercises.

If the patient will completely relax his muscles, calmly and quietly review the day's happenings in the evening exercise and concentrate upon a high ideal in the morning exercise, the nervousness will gradually disappear.

CHAPTER XX

ON CONDUCTING HEALING CENTERS

GENERAL SUGGESTIONS:

As Probationers in various places have banded themselves together to study Astro-Diagnosis and Astro-Therapy with a view to forming Healing Centers when they shall have become sufficiently grounded in these sciences, it may be well to give a few suggestions for the conduct of such centers.

In the first place we must remember that whatever is to be done is for Christ's sake, and devotional exercises at the commencement of classes are an absolute necessity in order to balance the intellectual side of the work. Let us remember that the Christ is now imprisoned in the earth for our sake, bearing the heavy burden of the earth so that we may have proper conditions for our evolution; that disease is the result of ignorance of cosmic laws, hence a retarding factor in evolution and therefore a cause of prolongation of the Christ's imprisonment; and that when we alleviate human suffering we are at the same time decreasing the suffering of Christ and hastening the day of His liberation.

Devotional exercises are a powerful means of putting us in tune with the Christ. Through them we gain an intuitional faculty whereby we feel the suffering of others, and at the same time we find the way to ease their pain as Parsifal did the cause of Amfortas' suffering when he was in the garden with Kundry and there realized how he might heal the stricken king. So first and foremost, let us have devotional exercised, reading from the Bible with reference to how Christ healed the sick and comforted the suffering. Perhaps a few comments to drive home the lesson, would be well.

Take THE IMITATION OF CHRIST, by Thomas a Kempis, or anything else of a thoroughly devotional nature, and then turn to the study of the human body, for a knowledge of anatomy is an absolute essential. The body is the temple for the indwelling Spirit, and as it is necessary for an architect to know how to prop up the pillars of a church, when the wear and tear of time have caused the foundation to crumble, so that new material may replace that which has decayed to make the edifice strong and useful again, so also must we know how to strengthen the various parts of the living temple with which we are to deal. There is a book called THE STORY OF

THE LIVING TEMPLE, by Rossiter, which treats of the body in a spiritual manner and will service admirably as an aid to a higher conception while using the ordinary textbooks.

When taking up a horoscope for analysis, be sure you do not use the figures for Probationers attending the meetings, or their close relatives. For just as students in a medical college often by suggestion develop the symptoms of the diseases they are studying, so also members of the class are apt to suffer from neglect of the above precaution. Moreover, when a Probationer is ill and applies to the Center for healing, he or she may not be admitted to the classes while in ill health, for it is absolutely impossible to avoid accidental mention of symptoms from which such a one may suffer, and thus the disease may be aggravated in this manner.

ADVICE TO HEALERS

If letters of fire that would burn themselves into the consciousness of the reader were obtainable, we would spare no effort to procure them for the purpose of warning students on some particular points in connection with the practice of Medical Astrology; these are:

Never tell a patient a discouraging fact.

Never tell him when impending crises are due.

Never predict sickness at a certain time.

Never, NEVER predict death.

It is a grave mistake, almost a crime, to tell sick persons anything discouraging, for it robs them of strength that should he husbanded with the utmost care to facilitate recovery. It is also wrong to suggest sickness to a well person, for it focuses the mind on a specific disease at a certain time, and such a suggestion is liable to cause sickness. It is a well-known fact that many students in medical colleges feel the symptoms of every disease they study, and suffer greatly in consequence of autosuggestion, but the idea of impending disease implanted by one in whom the victim has faith is much more dangerous. Therefore, it behooves the medical astrologer to be very cautious. If you cannot say something encouraging, be silent.

This warning applies with particular force when treating patients having Taurus or Virgo rising or the Sun or Moon in those signs. These positions predispose the mind to center on disease, often in a most unwarranted manner. The Taurean fears sickness to an almost insane degree, and prediction of disease is fatal to his nature. The Virgoans court disease, in order to gain sympathy, and though professing to long for recovery, they actually delight in probing the matter to the depths; they will plead ability to stand full knowledge and profess that it will help them; but if the practitioner allows himself to be enticed by their protestations, and does tell them, they wilt like a flower. They are the most difficult people to help in any case, and extra care should be taken not to aggravate their chances by admissions of the nature indicated. Some students have a morbid desire to know the time of their own death, and probe into this matter in a most unwarranted manner; but no matter how they may seek to deceive themselves there are very few who have the mental and moral stamina to live life in the same manner, if they knew with absolute certainty that on a certain date their earthly existence would be terminated. This is one of the points most wisely hidden until we are able to see on both sides of the veil, and we do wrong, no matter what our ground, to seek to wrest that knowledge from the horoscope.

In the past when our efforts in behalf of the sick were necessarily restricted to members on account of lack of help in the office the questions sometimes asked: "How may I help a sick friend?" Though we are now prepared to render aid from Headquarters to "whosoever will" some, it is important to impress upon probationers of the great opportunity which is theirs by virtue of the connection they have established with the Teacher. Healing is accomplished principally by Probationers who "live the life" under direction of the Elder Brothers; and application TO THEM, written with pen and ink, whether directed through Headquarters or to a Probationer, invariably evokes a response.

The Elder Brothers know how to use the law to the best advantage, but cannot work contrary to it nor do more than the material furnished them admits, physical sickness may be overcome by spiritual power, but a certain amount of this power is required. It is a law of physics that a number of coals must be heaped together and sufficient oxygen furnished in order to make a fire. Christ said, "Where two or three are gathered together in my name, there will I be among them."

Association of Probationers in Center of Healing furnishes the material in which the Elder Brothers may kindle the Spiritual Fire required to heal physical, moral, and mental ailments. Single-handed there is small change of doing good, but in numbers there is strength, particularly if all are fortified with a knowledge of diagnosis from the horoscope and how to apply treatment at propitious times.

HEALING SERVICE INAUGURATED:

On Holy Night the spiritual power in the Sun culminates, pouring out a benediction upon the air. From the 25th of December to the 25th of June the physical activities are in the ascendant, gradually gathering force which culminates at the Summer Solstice; and then blesses man physically with the things needed for his material sustenance. During that time the spiritual activities are difficult to inaugurate, and therefore we waited quietly until the turn recently, holding the first evening healing service on Tuesday, the 23rd of June (1914), at half past seven, when the Moon was in the cardinal sign of Cancer. And in the future a healing service will be held in the Pro-Ecclesia each week at that hour on a day when the Moon is in one of the cardinal signs. We decided to have these services that we might utilize the little Pro-Ecclesia to the very utmost, and thus earn the privilege of having the Ecclesia, too. This was approved by the Teacher, and he suggested that the healing service be held when the Moon is in the cardinal signs. But we want to go a step further in our efforts to secure efficiency; and this is where we want to add the help of every earnest student in The Rosicrucian Fellowship.

There is a passage in the ritual used at The Rosicrucian Fellowship services which says: "One coal cannot make a fire, but where a number of coals are gathered together the heat which is latent in each may be kindled into a flame emitting light and warmth. It is in obedience to the same law of Nature that we have gathered here tonight, that by massing our spiritual aspirations we may light and keep ablaze the beacon light of true spiritual fellowship." The power of numbers is insignificant in the world of physical existence, compared with the power of the same number in the spiritual realm. Here additions to the power of a community count as one, two, three, four, etc., but there the power increases in a proportion that might be likened to the square; two, four, eight, sixteen, etc., for the first twelve who attend a spiritual service. The thirteenth then would bring it up into another higher realm of the spiritual universe. For the sake of illustration, we may count the increase there by the power of three, nine, twenty-seven, etc., as so on. Thus you will see how important even the very weakest one among us may become WHEN IT IS A QUESTION OF MASSING OUR SPIRITUAL ASPIRATIONS. Nor can there by any questions of the powerful influence that will have on the sick.

To secure the help of all earnest students and give them the privilege of helping, we will publish in the Echoes each month the date on which the healing services will be held, and if each student will sit down in his or her own home at half past seven, directing their thoughts to Mt. Ecclesia, to the little Pro-Ecclesia, where the symbol of the Invisible Helpers will then be unveiled, the love, sympathy, and strength thus given these workers will enable them to do a much greater service for humanity; each one of course them having part in that work. The symbol of the Invisible Helpers upon which we concentrate at Mt. Ecclesia is a snow-white cross, with the seven red roses and a pure white one in the center; the usual stars (the rays), goes out from the cross, and the background is blue, the whole being beautifully illuminated, thus making it an apt emblem of the effulgence of that soul body wherein these workers travel. It will not be necessary to make corrections in time for your place of residence, because the Sun will gather all the aspirations as he goes along, and when the rays at the proper angle arrive at Mt. Ecclesia the influence directed here will certainly transmit itself and unite with our aspirations taking place at this time and help us in the work. (NOTE: The time of this healing service has since been changed to half past six.)

PART IV

"THERE IS NO DEATH"

CHAPTER XXI

THE REAL NATURE OF DEATH

Amid all the uncertainties which are the characteristics of this world, there is but one certainty--Death. At one time or another, after a short or long life, comes this termination to the material phase of our existence, which is a birth into a new world, as that which we term "birth" is, in the beautiful words of Wordsworth, a forgetting of the past.

Birth and death may therefore be regarded has the shifting of man's activity from one world to another, and it depends upon our own position whether we designate such a change birth or death. If he enters the world in which we live, we call it birth; if he leaves our plane of existence to enter another world, we call it death. To the individual concerned, however, the passage from one world to another is but as a removal to another city here; he LIVES, unchanged; only his exterior surroundings and condition are changed.

The passage from one world to another is often attended by more or less unconsciousness, like sleep, as Wordsworth says, and for the reason our consciousness may be fixed upon the world we have left. In infancy heaven lies about us in actual fact; children are all clairvoyant for a longer or shorter time after birth, and whoever passes out at death still beholds the material world for some time. If we pass out in the full vigor of physical manhood or womanhood, with strong times of family, friends, or other interests, the dense world will continue to attract our attention for a much longer time than if death occurred at a "ripe old age," when the earthy ties have been severed before the change we call death. This is on the same principle that the seed clings to the flesh of unripe fruit, while it is easily and cleanly detached from the ripe fruit. Therefore it is easier to die at an advanced age than in youth.

The unconsciousness which usually attends the change of the incoming spirit at birth, and the outgoing spirit at death, is due to our inability to adjust our focus instantly, and is similar to the difficulty we experience when passing from a darkened room to the street on a light, sunny day, or vice versa. Under those conditions some time elapses before we can distinguish objects about us; so with the newly born and the newly dead, both have to readjust their viewpoint to their new condition.

When the moment arrives which marks the completion of life in the physical world, the usefulness of the dense body has ended, and the Ego withdraws from it by way of the head, taking with it the mind and the desire body, as it does every night during sleep, but now the vital body is useless, so that, too, is withdrawn, and when the silver cord which united the higher to the lower vehicles snaps it can never be repaired.

We remember that the vital body is composed of ether, superimposed upon the dense bodies of plant, animal, and man during life. Ether is physical matter, and therefore has weight. The only reason why the scientists cannot weigh it is because they are unable to gather a quantity and put it on a scale. But when it leaves the dense body at death a diminution in weight will take place in every instance, showing that something having weight, yet invisible, leaves the dense body at that time.

Physical science knows that whatever the power which moves the heart, it does not come from without, but is inside the heart. The occult scientists sees a chamber in the left ventricle, near the apex, where a little atom swims in a sea of the highest ether. The force in that atom, like the forces of all other atoms, is THE UNDIFFERENTIATED LIFE OF GOD; without that force the mineral could not form matter into crystals, the plant, animal, and human kingdoms would be unable to form their bodies. The deeper we go the plainer it becomes to us how fundamentally true it is that in God we live, more, and have our being.

That atom is called the "seed atom." The force within it moves the heart and keeps the organism alive. All the other atoms in the whole body must vibrate in tune with this atom. The forces of the seed-atom have been immanent in every dense body every possessed by the particular Ego to whom it is attached, and upon its plastic tablet are inscribed all the experiences of that particular Ego in all its lives. When we return to God, when we shall have become one in God once more, that record, which is peculiarity God's record, will still remain, and thus we shall retain our individuality. Our experiences we transmute into faculties; the evil is transmuted into good and the good we retain as power for higher good, but THE RECORD of the experiences is OF God and IN God; in the most intimate sense.

The "silver cord" which unites the higher and lower vehicles terminates at the seed atom in the heart. When material life comes to an end in the natural manner the forces in the seed atom disengage themselves, pass outward along the pneumogastric nerve, the back of the head and along the silver cord, together with the higher vehicles. It is this rupture in the heart which marks physical death, but the connecting silver cord is not broken at once, in some cases not for several days.

CHAPTER XXII

EFFECTS OF SUICIDE

When the Ego is coming down to rebirth it descends through the Second Heaven. There it is helped by the Creative Hierarchies to build an archetype for its coming body, and it instills into that archetype a life that will last for a certain number of years. These archetypes are hollow spaces and they have a singing, vibratory motion which draws the material of the Physical World into them and sets all the atoms in the body vibrating in tune with a little atom that is in the heart, called the seed-atom, which, like a tuning fork, gives the pitch to all the rest of the material in the body. At the time when the full life has been lived on the earth the vibrations in the archetype cease, the seed-atom is withdrawn, the dense body goes to decay and the desire body, wherein the Ego functions in Purgatory and in the First Heaven, takes upon itself the shape of the physical body. Then the man commences his work of expiating his evil habits and deeds in Purgatory and assimilating the good of his life in the First Heaven.

The foregoing describes the ordinary conditions when the course of nature is undisturbed, but the case of the suicide is different. He has taken away the seed-atom, but the hollow archetype still keeps on vibrating. Therefore he feels as if he were hollowed out and experiences a gnawing feeling inside that can be best likened to the pangs of intense hunger. Material for the building of a dense body is all around him, but seeing that he lacks the gauge of the seed atom, it is impossible for him to assimilate that matter and build it into a body. This dreadful hollowed- out feeling lasts as long as his ordinary life should have lasted. Thus the Law of Cause and Effect teaches him that it is wrong to play truant from the school of life and that it cannot be done with impunity. Then in the next life, when difficulties beset his path, he will remember the sufferings of the past which resulted from suicide and go through the experience that makes for his soul growth.

It is curious that the commission of suicide in one life and the consequent post-mortem suffering during the time when the archetype still exists often generate in such people a morbid fear of death tin the next life; so that when the event actually occurs in the ordinary course of life, they seem frantic after they leave the body and so anxious to get back to the Physical World again that they frequently commit the crime of obsession in the most foolish and unthinking manner.

CHAPTER XXIII

CAUSES OF DEATH DURING INFANCY

When a man passes out a death, he takes with him the mind, desire body, and vital body the latter being the storehouse of the pictures of his past life. And during the three and one-half days following death these pictures are etched into the desire body to form the basis of man's life in Purgatory and the First Heaven where the evil is expurgated and the good assimilated. The experience of the life itself is forgotten, as we have forgotten the process of learning to write, but have retained the faculty. So the cumulative extract of all his experiences, both during past earth lives and past existences in Purgatory and the various heavens, are retained by the man and form his stock in trade in the next birth. The pains he has sustained speak to him as the voice of conscience, the good he had done gives him a more and more altruistic character.

Now, when the three and a half days immediately following death are spent by man under conditions of peace and quiet, he is able to concentrate much more upon the etching of his past life and the imprint upon the desire body will be deeper than if he is disturbed by the hysterical lamentations of his relatives or from other causes. He will then experience a much keener feeling for either good or bad in Purgatory and in the First Heaven, and in after lives that keen feeling will speak to him with no unmistakable voice; but where the lamentations of relatives take away his attention or where a man passes out by accident, perhaps in a crowded street, in a train wreck, theatre fire, or under other harrowing circumstances, there will, of course, be no opportunity for him to concentrate properly; neither can he concentrate on a battle field if he is slain there, and yet it would not be just that he would lose the experience of his life on account of passing out in such an untoward manner, so that the Law of Cause and Effect provides a compensation.

We usually think that when a child is born it is born and that is an end to it; but as during the period of gestation the dense body is shielded from the impact of the outside world by being placed within the protecting womb of the mother until it has arrived at sufficient maturity to meet the outside conditions, so are also the vital body, desire body, and mind in a state of gestation and are born at later periods because they have not had as long an evolution behind them as the dense body. Therefore, it takes a longer time for them to arrive at a sufficient state of maturity to become individualized. The vital body is born at the seventh year, when the period of excessive growth marks its advent. The desire body is born at the time of puberty, the fourteenth year, and the mind is born at twenty-one, when the child is said to have become a man or woman.....to have reached majority.

That which has not been quickened cannot die, and so when a child dies before the birth of the desire body it passes out into the invisible world into the First Heaven. It cannot ascend into the Second and Third Heaven because the mind and desire body are not born and will not die, so it simply waits in the First Heaven until a new opportunity for embodiment offers, and where it has died in its previous life under the before-mentioned harrowing circumstances by accident or upon the battle field or where the lamentations of relatives rendered it impossible for it to gain as deep an impression of evil committed and the good accomplished as would have been the case had it died in peace, it is instructed when it has died in the next life as a child in the effects of passions and desires so that it learns the lessons then which it should have learned in the purgatorial life had it remained undisturbed. It is then reborn with the proper development of conscience so that it may continue its evolution.

As in the past man has been exceedingly warlike and not at all careful of the relatives who passed out at death because of his ignorance, holding wakes over those who died in bed, which were few, perhaps, compared to those who died on the battle field, there must necessarily on that account be an enormous amount of infant mortality, but as humanity arrives at a better understanding and realizes that we never so much our brother's keeper as when he is passing out of this life and that we can help him enormously by being quiet and prayerful, so also will infant mortality cease to exist on such a large scale as at present.

CHAPTER XXIV

PROPER CARE OF THE DECEASED

The vital body is the vehicle of sense-perception. As it remains with the body of feeling (the desire body) and the etheric cord connects them with the discarded dense body, it will be evident that until the cord is severed there must be a certain amount of feeling experienced by the Ego when its dense body is molested. Thus, it causes pain when the blood is extracted and embalming fluid injected, when the body is opened for post-mortem examination, and when the body is cremated.

A case was told the writer in which a surgeon amputated three toes from a living person under anesthetics. He threw the severed toes into a bright coal fire, and immediately the patient commenced to scream, for the rapid disintegration of the material toes caused an equally rapid disintegration of the etheric toes, which were connected with the higher vehicles. In like manner molestations affect the discarnate Spirit from a few hours to three and a half days after death. Then all connection is severed and the body begins to decay.

Therefore great care should be taken not to cause the passing Spirit discomfort by such measures. Quiet and prayer are of enormous benefit at that time, and if we love the departed Spirit wisely we shall be able to earn its lasting gratitude by following the above instructions.

A word should be spoken in regard to the treatment of dying persons who suffer unspeakable agony in many cases through the mistaken kindness of friends. More suffering is caused by administering stimulants to the dying than perhaps in any other way. It is not hard to pass out of the body, but stimulants have the effect of throwing the departing Ego back into its body with the force of a catapult, to experience anew the sufferings from which it was just escaping. Departing souls have often complained to investigators, and one such person said that he had not suffered as much in all his life as he did while kept from dying for many hours. The only rational way is to leave Nature to take its course when it is seen that the end is inevitable.

Another and more far-reaching sin against the passing Spirit is to give vent to loud crying or lamentation in or near the death chamber. Just subsequent to its release and from a few hours to a few days afterwards, the Ego is engaged upon a matter of the utmost importance; a great deal of the value of the past life depends upon the attention given to it by the passing Spirit. If distracted by the sobs and lamentations of loved ones, it will lose much, but if strengthened by prayer and helped by silence, much future sorrow to all concerned may be avoided. We are never so much our brother's keeper as when he is passing through this Gethsemane, and it is one of our greatest opportunities for serving him and laying up heavenly treasure for ourselves.

We have studied the phenomenon of birth, and have evolved a SCIENCE OF BIRTH. We have qualified obstetricians and trained nurses to minister in the best possible manner to both mother and child to make them comfortable, but we are sadly, very sadly, in need of a SCIENCE OF DEATH. When a child is coming into the world we bustle about in an intelligent endeavor; when a lifelong friend is about to leave us we stand helplessly about, ignorant of how to aid; worse than all, we bungle, and cause suffering instead of helping.

We have stated that the vital body is the storehouse of both the conscience and subconscious memory; upon the vital body is branded indelibly every act and experience of the past life, as the scenery upon an exposed photographic plate. When the Ego has withdrawn it from the dense body, the whole life, as registered by the subconscious memory, is laid open to the eye of the mind. It is the partial loosening of the vital body which causes a drowning person to see his whole past life, but then it is only like a flash, preceding unconsciousness; the silver cord remains intact, or there could be no resuscitation. In the case of a Spirit passing out at death, the movement is slower; the man stands as a spectator while the pictures succeed one another from death to birth, so that he sees the first happenings just prior to death then the years of manhood and womanhood unroll themselves; youth, childhood and infancy follow, until it terminates at birth. The man, however, has no feeling about them at that time, the object is merely to etch the panorama into the desire body, which is the seat of feeling, and from that impress the feeling will be realized when the Ego enters the Desire World, but we may note there that THE INTENSITY

OF FEELING REALIZED DEPENDS UPON THE LENGTH OF TIME CONSUMED IN THE PROCESS OF ETCHING, AND THE ATTENTION GIVEN THERETO BY THE MAN. IF HE WAS UNDISTURBED FOR A LONG PERIOD, A DEEP CLEAR-CUT IMPRESS WILL BE MADE UPON THE DESIRE BODY. HE WILL FEEL THE WRONG HE DID MORE KEENLY IN PURGATORY, AND BE MORE ABUNDANTLY STRENGTHENED IN HIS GOOD QUALITIES IN HEAVEN, and though the experience will be lost in a future life, THE FEELINGS WILL REMAIN, as the "still small voice." Where the feelings have been strongly indented upon the desire body of an Ego, this voice will speak in no vague and uncertain terms. It will impel him beyond gainsaying, forcing him to desist from that which caused him pain in the life before and compel him to yield to that which is good. Therefore the panorama passed BACKWARDS, so that the Ego sees first the effects, and then the underlying causes.

When the body is buried, the vital body disintegrates slowly at the same time as the dense body, so that when, for instance, an arm has decayed in the grave, the etheric arm of the vital body which hovers over the grave also disappears, and so on until the last vestige of the body is gone. But where cremation is performed the vital body disintegrates at once, and as that is the storehouse of the pictures of the past life, which are being etched upon the desire body to form the basis of life in Purgatory and the First Heaven, this would be a great calamity where cremation is performed before the three and a half days are passed. Unless help were given, the passing Spirit could not hold it together. And that is part of the work that is done by the Invisible Helpers for humanity. Sometimes they are assisted by nature spirits and others detailed by the Creative Hierarchies or leaders of humanity. There is also a loss where one is cremated before the silver cord has been broken naturally, the imprint upon the desire body is never as deep as it would otherwise have been, and this has an effect upon future lives, for the deeper the imprint of the last life upon the desire body, the keener the sufferings in Purgatory for the ill committed and the keener also the pleasure in the First Heaven which results from the good deeds of the last life. It is these pains and pleasures of our past lives that are what we call conscience, so that where we have lost in suffering we lose also the realization of wrong which is to deter us in future lives from committing the same mistakes again. Therefore, the effects of the premature cremation are very far reaching.

As to what determines the length of the panorama, we remember that it was the collapse of the vital body which forced the higher vehicles to withdraw, so after death, when the vital body collapses, the Ego has to withdraw, and thus the panorama comes to an end. The duration of the panorama depends, therefore, upon the time the person could remain awake if necessary. Some people can remain awake only a few hours, others can endure for a few days, depending upon the strength of their vital body.

When the Ego has left the vital body, the latter gravitates back to the dense body, remaining hovering above the grave, decaying as the dense body does, and it is indeed a noisome sight to the clairvoyant to pass through a cemetery and behold all those vital bodies whose state of decay clearly indicates the state of decomposition of the remains in the grave. If there were more clairvoyants, incineration would soon be adopted as a measure of protection to our feelings, if not for sanitary reasons.

As the interest and belief in a life after death becomes more universal, the necessity for a scientific method for the care of those who are passing into the higher life will be impressed upon the people, and we shall then have nurses, doctors, and ministers who are versed in the science of death as well as in the science of birth. The Spirit will then be surrounded by love and peace at the time of passing. It will also have a deeper and clearer record with which to begin its life work in its new state.

CHAPTER XXV

HOW TO HELP THOSE WHO HAVE PASSED ON

When the Ego comes into the Physical World, it is in one sense a cause for rejoicing, as we rejoice at the birth of a child, for this world affords us experience and material for soul growth. Looking at if from another point of view, however, when the Ego comes into this world and enters the prison house of the dense body, it is in the most limited condition imaginable, and to rejoice at the time the child is born and lament when it is liberated by death, is in reality analogous to rejoicing when a friend is put in jail and giving way to hysterical lamentation when he is liberated.

Furthermore, our duties to our dear ones who have passed away from the earth life are not ended when they have severed the physical ties. We have a responsibility to them beyond the grave. Our attitude after the death of our loved ones continues to affect them, for they do not usually leave their accustomed places right away. Many stay in or near the home for a number of months after they have left the body and can feel conditions there even more keenly than when in earth life. If we sigh, mourn, and groan for them we transfer to them the gloom we ourselves carry about us or else we bind them to home in efforts to cheer us. In either case we are a hindrance and a stumbling black in the way of their spiritual progress, and while this may be forgiven in those who are ignorant of the facts concerning life and death, people who have studied the Rosicrucian Philosophy or kindred teachings are incurring a very grave responsibility when they indulge in such practices.

We are well aware that custom used to demand the wearing of mourning and that people were not considered respectable if they did not put on a sable garb as a token of their grief. Fortunately, times are changing and a more enlightened view is being taken of the matter. The transition to the other world is quite serious enough in itself, involving as it does a process of adjustment to strange conditions all around, and the passing spirit is further hampered by the sorrow and anguish of the dear ones whom it continues to see about itself, when it finds them surrounded by a cloud of black gloom, clothed in garments of the same color and nursing their sorrow for months or years, the effect cannot be anything but depressing.

How much better the attitude of those who have learned the Rosicrucian Teachings and have taken them to heart. Their attitude is cheerful, helpful, hopeful, and encouraging. The selfish grief at the loss is suppressed in order that the passing spirit may receive all the encouragement possible. Usually the survivors in the family dress in white at the funeral and a cheerful, genial spirit prevails throughout. The thought of the survivors is not, "What shall I do now that I have lost him? All the world seems empty for me." It is, "I hope that he may find himself rights under the new conditions as quickly as possible and that he will not grieve at the thought of leaving us behind." We pray earnestly for his welfare and that he may learn the lessons of this life thoroughly in his experiences in Purgatory and the First Heaven.

Thus, by the good will, intelligence, unselfishness, and love of the remaining friends the passing Spirit is enabled to enter the new conditions under much more favorable circumstances, and we cannot do better than to spread this teaching as widely as possible. It is our loss if we are blind to the superphysical realms, but to all who will take the trouble to awaken their latent faculties, the opening of the proper sense is but a matter of time. When that time comes we shall see the so-called "dead" are all about us, and that, in fact, "there is no death," as John McCreery says in the following beautiful poem:

There is no death. The stars go down

To rise upon another shore,

And bright in heaven's jeweled crown

They shine forevermore.

There is no death. The forest leaves

Convert to life the viewless air;

The rocks disorganize to feed

The hungry moss they bear.

There is no death. The dust we tread

Shall change beneath the summer showers

To golden grain or mellow fruit,

Or rainbow-tinted flowers.

There is no death. The leaves may fall,

    The flowers may fade and pass away--

They only wait through wintry hours

    The warm, sweet breath of May.

There is no death, although we grieve

    When beautiful familiar forms

That we have learned to love are torn

    From our embracing arms.

Although with bowed and breaking heart,

    With sable garb and silent tread

We bear their senseless dust to rest

    And say that they are dead--

They are not dead. They have but passed

    Beyond the mists that blind us here

Into the new and larger life

    Of that serener sphere.

They have but dropped their robe of clay

    To put a shining raiment on;

They have not wandered far away,

They are not 'lost' or 'gone.'

Though unseen to the mortal eye,

They still are here and love us yet;

The dear ones they have left behind

They never do forget.

Sometimes upon our fevered brow

We feel their touch, a breath of balm;

Our spirit sees them, and our hearts

Grow comforted and calm.

Yes, even near us, though unseen,

Our dear, immortal spirits tread--

For all God's boundless Universe

Is Life--there are no dead.

www.ingramcontent.com/pod-product-compliance
Lightning Source LLC
Chambersburg PA
CBHW070048210526
45170CB00012B/619